Weigh Every Day

*Achieve lifetime weight loss
with a stress-free daily weigh-
in and personal food rules*

Sylvia Moestl Vasilik

ISBN 978-1-7341663-0-9 (ebook)

ISBN 978-1-7341663-1-6 (paperback)

Published by Fluid Progress Press

Visit **WeighEveryDay.com**

v. 86

Note to Readers

The anecdotes in this book are used to illustrate common problems and issues that I have encountered and do not necessarily portray specific people or situations. No real names have been used.

The information in this book is the opinion of the author and is based on the author's observations and experiences. It is intended only as an informational guide to health issues. It is sold with the understanding that the author is not engaged in rendering medical, health, psychological or any other kind of personal professional services or therapy in the book. This book should not be used to diagnose or treat any medical condition.

The author and publisher specifically disclaim all responsibility for any liability, loss, or risk, personal or otherwise, which is incurred as a consequence, directly or indirectly, of the use and application of any of the contents of this book. This book is not intended to replace or conflict with the advice given to you by your doctor. The final decision concerning medical care should be made between you and your doctor.

Contents

INTRODUCTION

If you're reading this book, I'm going to make a few assumptions. One is that you want to lose weight—that one is obvious.

The other assumption is that you're open to unconventional ideas.

How do I know this? Because the title of the book, Weigh Every Day, tells you the first principle of the book. Which is, of course, that you should weigh yourself—every single day. And weighing yourself every day goes against a lot of "common sense" wisdom that's been pushed for decades. The accepted wisdom is that you should weigh yourself at most once a week. Many people say you should even throw away your scale entirely.

But still—you picked up this book. So, you must be a person that's willing to at least consider an idea that's not mainstream. That's a good thing, because the advice to weigh yourself every day is just the first of some of the unconventional advice I have.

✳✳✳

Why did I write this book? I'm not a medical doctor. I'm not an obesity researcher. I don't have a degree in nutrition. My career is in computer programming, for crying out loud. And my personal story of weight loss is not a dramatic "How I lost 100 pounds in a year", or anything like that.

Instead, it's a much more ordinary, mundane story. But it reflects what has happened to most people in the US over the past 30 or so years. It's a story of gradual, slow, weight gain, with a few periods of weight loss. There were also some periods where my weight was stable—but with a lot of stress and effort. And finally, a period where my weight has been stable at a reasonable level, with little effort, and without stress. And that's what many of us are aiming for—staying healthy and keeping our weight at a reasonable level, without "dieting", without meal plans, and without anxiety.

A friend of mine, Ryan, has been trying to lose weight for a while. He was skeptical when I told him I was writing this book. He said, "You haven't ever had a *serious* weight problem. How can you know what it's like?"

It's true—I've never been clinically obese, or lost huge, dramatic amounts of weight. When it comes to weight, I'm an average person, living in the same food environment that we all live in. And just like the average person, I was slowly and steadily gaining weight.

But then I discovered some principles that helped me solve my weight problem. And I believe they can help you, too.

✳✳✳

Earlier, I wrote that I'm a computer programmer. Specifically, I work with data. For many years now, I've programmed databases, analyzed data, and studied data trends. That analysis and research mindset has helped me in my work on this book.

2

In my research for this book, I've reviewed more than 60 books on weight management, dieting, and obesity. These have been books of all sorts—from academic ones, heavy on statistics, to memoirs written by people who lost a tremendous amount of weight, to diet books with strange themes ("The Aztec Diet: Chia Power: The Superfood that Gets You Skinny and Keeps You Healthy").

Many of these books had alarming statistics in them, on the percentage of the population in the United States that was overweight or obese. As I'm writing this book, in 2019, the latest published statistics are from 2016. They show that in the United States, more than 71% of the population is overweight or obese.

But many of the books that I reviewed had different and lower numbers—60%, 66%, etc. When I looked carefully at them, though, it became clear why the numbers were off. It was the *older* books that had the lower numbers. Back in the early 1970s, the percentage of people who were overweight and obese was 47%. It's been going up slowly and steadily. Around the year 2000, it was 64%. Recently (2015-2016), it hit 71%.

Where is it going to end? Will the percentage of people that are overweight or obese be like the percentage of smokers? That number is going down steadily. In the 1960s, more than 40% of the population of the United States smoked, but in 2015 it was only 15%.

Or will the percentage keep on going up and up, until it becomes rare to see someone that's not overweight or obese?

Personally, I don't see signs that the obesity epidemic is changing direction soon. I don't have a crystal ball, but the numbers show that our society is becoming *more* obese, not less.

But this book is not targeted to "society". I don't have recommendations for government policies like subsidizing fruits and vegetables, or taxing soda.

Instead, it's a book for one person—you. I want to help you lose weight and keep it off, despite living in a world that encourages the exact opposite. Even though most of the population is getting heavier and heavier—you don't need to. You can still lose weight. And in this book, I share some of the principles that I have discovered over the years, about what works, and what doesn't work.

✳✳✳

When I was about 30 years old, I noticed that my weight had been going up, slowly. Before then, I didn't have a scale, and never weighed myself. But I bought a scale, and started weighing myself every day. The awareness caused by stepping on the scale every day stopped that slow weight gain, and I lost some pounds.

After the birth of my first child, I had a hard time losing about 15 pounds of stubborn baby weight. Months and months went by, and those pounds just wouldn't come off. So, I got hard-core. To me, that meant counting calories. I bought a food scale and installed an app to log my food. Absolutely everything I ate was weighed and measured. I learned two things from that experience:

- Counting calories *works*. If you're accurate, take the time and effort to do it right, and set the right calorie targets, you *will* lose weight.
- Counting calories takes a lot of work! Every single bite needs to be logged. It's okay for a short time, but not many people could make it a lifetime habit.

4

My weight was not a problem for a while after this. But slowly, over the years, the weight started creeping up again. I noticed it mainly when returning from vacations. It was normal for me to gain a few pounds on a vacation, then lose it in a week or two. But that stopped happening. The weight that I gained during vacations stuck around.

That was frustrating. I knew that calorie counting worked, but I also knew that it didn't make sense, for fighting this type of very slow weight gain. I knew that whatever I did needed to be something that I could do for a lifetime—and I couldn't count calories for a lifetime. But I also hated the idea that I was going to steadily, inevitably, gain weight.

✱✱✱

Friends of mine were having similar problems. They went on all kinds of weight loss programs. But some of these programs pushed food rules that I thought were absolutely crazy. Rules like not eating foods like green peas, corn on the cob, and sweet potatoes. Some programs had restrictions on weighing yourself, and asked you to promise to weigh yourself only at their office.

These rules seemed like they would be useless over the long term—even counterproductive. But I didn't really have any alternatives that I thought were better. Since calorie counting had worked for me, as a short-term strategy, I thought maybe I could do an easier version of that. For instance, instead of actually weighing and measuring everything, just taking a photo of everything I ate.

But I never even started that one. The thought of photographing everything I ate seemed like it would be annoying and weird, and impossible to keep up for a lifetime.

I brainstormed a few other ideas. I did lots of research. And I learned that the average American is much heavier now than 50 years ago, and why that is. I uncovered some of the dangers of today's food environment. I explored some of the food hazards that you need to limit, or avoid completely, to lose weight and keep it off.

And finally, I figured out the personal food rules that work for me, that help me lose weight and keep it off, without much effort or thought.

My food rules and guidelines won't be the same as yours. But the principles that you use to develop them are universal.

Weighing yourself daily is the first and most important strategy for managing your weight in today's food environment. It keeps you honest and grounded in reality. It's important enough that it's in the title of the book, and I've focused multiple chapters on it.

Weighing yourself every day is important, but it's not enough. You also need to understand what foods and food habits are hazardous, and which rules and guidelines can help you avoid them. This is not something that happens overnight. It's a slow, step-by-step process. But once you figure it out, it's yours for life.

I hope that with this book, I can convince you of a few ideas. These ideas are:

- **The rising tide of obesity we're living with is new, and caused by a mismatch**. This mismatch is between a strong biological urge to eat whenever delicious food is available—and the fact that today, delicious food is always available.

- **Many of the foods that are causing us to gain weight are not traditional foods**, that people have eaten for thousands of years. Instead, they're new foods, developed in labs, and designed to be as addictive as possible.
- **Weighing yourself daily is the easiest, healthiest habit you can develop**. It's a simple, straightforward way of getting feedback on your eating habits. And weighing yourself can be anxiety-free.
- **Abstinence can be much easier than moderation.** Moderation—just eating less of the food that you want to limit—can be very difficult. And abstinence—never eating certain foods—can be much easier. By reducing choices, abstinence can reduce food cravings and obsessions.
- **Food rules, personalized to meet your needs and lifestyle**, are one of the most effective ways of losing weight and maintaining your weight loss. Food rules can make good food habits automatic. Food rules can be designed so that you can keep them up for life.

Many, many people struggle with their weight. This is happening because the current food environment is constantly pushing us to overeat. Food advertising, and the sight and smells of tempting foods surround us, and are very powerful.

But ideas are powerful, too. By arming yourself with these ideas, and translating them into action, you can achieve the lifetime weight loss you're looking for.

7

For weight charts and other resources, blog posts, and contact information, please visit my website:

WeighEveryDay.com

THE HISTORY OF OBESITY

Throughout history, people have lived with famine and hunger. Now, we have abundance—which can be a double-edged sword.

As a nation, we have been transformed, in just a few decades. Most of us are not "normal" weight anymore. We're overweight or obese.

These are the facts, and there's no scientific debate about them at all. The obesity rate has jumped dramatically.

But here's what's also happening. People are forgetting that things were different, a few decades ago. If they're younger, perhaps they never knew it. This huge shift, this enormous jump in the number of people who are overweight or obese, is not noticed. And the factors causing it are not mentioned.

Here's what people do know. They know that they, as individuals, want to lose weight. Often, they blame themselves for having gained weight, and having a hard time losing it.

I'm here to tell you that it's important to understand why most people have gotten so much heavier. The reasons behind the obesity epidemic *matter*. They matter a lot. And understanding these reasons is critical for you, at a very personal level.

Why is this understanding so important? Some people don't think it is. Here's what they say:

Who cares why most of us are so overweight now? This historical stuff is a waste of time. Let's forget about all that, and get to the details—meal plans, recipes, and how many pounds I'll lose every week!

This reaction is very common. People are impatient, they want to get on with it, and fix their problems.

But knowing *why* we've gained so much weight is essential. Understanding how our food environment has changed in the past 30, 50, and 100 years is critical when you're trying to lose weight permanently. Because it's not a flaw or a problem with just one individual person (like "I just have no willpower"). That wouldn't explain why society as a whole, in most of the world, has become so much heavier.

No, the problem is that there's an enemy out there, that's actively pushing you towards weight gain. And that's what we'll learn about in this chapter. There have been many serious problems in human history—war, famine, epidemics, and diseases of all kinds. But this

10

problem, the dramatic explosion in obesity, has never happened before. And when you have a problem this dramatic, and completely new in history, you *must* understand why the problem is happening.

Say, for instance, that your car isn't working. You're in a parking lot, and can't start your car. When this happens, you need to know *why* it happened. You need to know, so you can figure out what to do next.

Do you need to:

- Dig out the jumper cables from the trunk, because the battery is dead?
- Call a friend to bring you some gas, because your tank is empty?

If you don't know *why* your car stopped running, you're going to waste time and energy, trying to solve the wrong problem. Knowing what really caused the problem is critical to fixing it. This applies to the problem of why your car is not running. And it also applies to the worldwide obesity problem.

To be clear, this is not a book about how to change society, or fix it in any way. It's a book for you, personally. For you to figure out how to lose weight, and keep it off for a lifetime.

So how does understanding the *cause* of our massive weight gain actually help you? It helps you because to lose weight, you need to change something. And that change needs to be based on an understanding of the root causes of obesity.

After you've learned more about why we've gained so much weight, you'll have a much better understanding of why weighing yourself daily is so important. And you'll be ahead of the game in figuring out which other food habits you should change, and how food rules can help you do this. Understanding why we—as a society—got so much heavier in the past decades can help you—personally—figure out how best to lose weight and keep it off.

Food throughout history was scarce— famine and hunger were common

Famine refers to a lack of food, because of drought, war, or other causes. Throughout history, humans have faced famine again and again. Famine means that a significant percentage of the population will die.

Many of our sources of recorded history mention famine again and again. Here are some Bible quotes about famine:

The seven years of plenty that occurred in the land of Egypt came to an end, and the seven years of famine began to come, as Joseph had said.
—Genesis 41:53

On the ninth day of the fourth month the famine was so severe in the city that there was no food for the people of the land
—2 Kings 25:3.

These are just a few of many dozens of quotes in the Bible, mentioning the famines that have occurred in recorded history. And fairy tales, at least in their original versions, also had many references to famine and hunger. Here's a famous story, in which famine is part of the plot:

Next to a great forest lived a poor woodcutter with his wife and his two children. The boy's name was Hansel and the girl was Gretel. The woodcutter had but little to eat, and once, when a great famine came to the land, he could no longer provide even their daily bread.

One evening as he was lying in bed worrying about his problems, he sighed and said to his wife, "What is to become of us? How can we feed our children when we have nothing for ourselves?"

Answered the woman. "Early tomorrow morning we will take the two children out into the thickest part of the woods, make a fire for them, and give each of them a little piece of bread, then leave them by themselves and go off to our work. They will not find their way back home, and we will be rid of them."

"No, woman," said the man. "I will not do that. How could I bring myself to abandon my own children alone in the woods? Wild animals would soon come and tear them to pieces."

"Oh, you fool," she said, "then all four of us will starve."

✳✳✳

The story of Hansel and Gretel is often sanitized now. But in the original versions, it's very clear that the two small children were sent out into the woods because there was a famine, and the parents had no food.

One of the greatest famines in recent Western European history is the Irish Potato Famine of the 1840s. Small farmers were dependent on potatoes for most of their food, and when the potato crop failed completely it was a disaster. More than 1 million people died, and many more were forced away from their homes in search of food.

✳✳✳

So, why am I bringing up all these stories of famine and hunger?

My point is this—in earlier times, hunger was part of most people's lives. Famine and hunger, the type of hunger that could lead to starvation, was something that our ancestors experienced regularly. Our ancestors survived because they had a very strong drive to search for food, and eat what was available, especially if it was high calorie.

It's a simple story. Those with a strong drive to eat, those that had built up some extra fat around the middle—they would survive. The others would not survive, and would not have children.

We are all descendants of the survivors. This means that through our genetic heritage, because of the thousands of generations who *survived* the famines, we have very powerful urges. These urges are pushing us to eat. They're encouraging us to build up some fat, to help us survive the upcoming famine.

The problem now, of course, is that there is no upcoming famine for most of us. Gradually, we achieved food abundance through improved farming techniques, and advances in food storage like canning and freezing. And all of these combined to make severe hunger and malnutrition a thing of the past.

Food now—tasty, cheap, and everywhere

Famines are—in most parts of the world—a thing of the past. But our bodies and our biological urges haven't changed. We still have a food drive that encourages us to eat as much high-calorie food as we can, whenever it's available. But what happens when it's always available? When we're constantly surrounded by convenient, delicious food—instead of simple foods, in limited quantities?

What happens is exactly what you'd expect. People gain weight, tremendous amounts of weight.

✳✳✳

The increase in obesity started very slowly, in the first part of the last century, but by the 1980s, weight gain began to accelerate dramatically.

Katherine Flegal was a scientist at the Center for Disease Control. In the early 1990s, while reviewing numbers from a massive federal government survey of health and nutrition, she realized that a dramatic change was occurring. The percentage of people who were over the normal weight—in other words, in the overweight and obese category—had gone up substantially in the 1980s. And it continued to rise over the next few decades.

Statistics from the Center for Disease Control show that between 1960 and 2016, we went from 44 percent overweight or obese, to 71 percent. And most of the change occurred in the obese category, instead of the overweight category. About the same percentage were overweight, but the number of people who were either obese or extremely obese went from 13 percent to 40 percent.

***

This weight gain occurred across the board. Both men and women, all races, all ages, gained lots of weight. Children weighed much more, and were entering adulthood much heavier than in previous generations.

Did this change take place only in the United States? No, it did not. The United States was the trailblazer in dramatic weight gain, but other countries followed. People got much heavier all over the world. In most countries that tracked health statistics, the records show that people gained large amounts of weight during this time. And this process is continuing.

These increases in body weight can cause serious, life-altering problems. People who've gained large amounts of weight have a much higher risk for diabetes, high blood pressure, heart disease, strokes, many types of cancer, and sleep apnea. Their joints hurt. They have problems fitting in seats in airplanes. They move around slowly and creakily.

Life expectancy, over the past century, had increased dramatically due to vaccines, improved hygiene, and medical advances. But no longer. Recently, life expectancy has actually *fallen* in the United States. This is a stunning setback.

✳✳✳

Why has this dramatic change in our weight occurred? Why did we gain so much weight? Did we become gluttons over the past decades? Did we lose all our willpower? Did our genetics, or hormones or something else inside our bodies change dramatically, that we gained so much weight?

The answer to all these questions is *no*. No, we didn't lose our willpower or become gluttons. Our genes did not change dramatically. The answer is much simpler.

Our food environment changed.

The amount of food we're surrounded by daily increased drastically. The number of times a day that we're exposed to food increased as well.

And most importantly, the *types of food* we're surrounded by changed. They changed dramatically, and in a way that makes us eat much, much more.

✳✳✳

Knowing more, rather than less, is always a good idea. And understanding the history of our food environment, and the dramatic changes that have taken place recently, is no exception. Knowledge is power.

But there's a specific reason that I'm going to be focusing on these changes. The reason is that understanding the changes that have occurred helps you figure out how to fight them. We're going to learn how our food environment changed, and how these changes have caused the epidemic of obesity.

After we learn this, it'll be easier for you to decide what will help you, personally. You can learn how to change your reaction to the toxic food environment, and develop your own habits and rules to combat it.

✱✱✱

Let's summarize the food environment that existed throughout most of history. It looked like this:

- Not much food in general. If you wasted food, you went hungry.
- Occasionally, almost no food (famine and hunger)
- A very limited variety of food
- Food was made by you or your family. Almost no processed food or restaurants
- Food was much more basic and less processed. Instead of Honey Nut Cheerios breakfast cereal, there was oatmeal

It sounds bleak, doesn't it? Always living on the edge, close to hunger?

That's why our ancestors worked hard to make food easier to come by. And especially over the past 100 years or so, they were very successful. So successful that we now have the problems of obesity instead of hunger.

What's our food environment like today? For every aspect of the food environment listed above, we have the *exact opposite*. For most people in the United States, it looks like this:

- Extreme abundance of food

- No famine or hunger
- Tremendous variety of food
- Most food is conveniently pre-processed and ready to eat, or eaten in restaurants
- Food is engineered to be addictive

Obviously, famine is a bad thing, and having enough food is a good thing. Nobody would argue that. But all these changes in our food environment have caused massive changes in our eating habits. We eat far, far more than we did before.

Hyperpalatable foods

There wouldn't be much overeating if we only had simple foods around. Take foods like plain, cooked oatmeal, or fresh apples. Many people love oatmeal and apples, but very few would eat too much of them.

There was a famous slogan on Lay's potato chips back in the 1960s; "Betcha can't just eat one". Well, that does not apply to carrot sticks. I can easily just eat one or two, and be perfectly happy.

But oatmeal, apples, and carrots sticks are *not* the foods that surround us daily, and tempt us constantly.

Here's a quote from the restaurant chain TGI Fridays, about how tempting their menus is:

This isn't about grabbing a bite. It's about a bite grabbing you. 'Cause when Friday's gets hold of your appetite, we're not letting go. We are going to bring on the flavor til your taste buds explode like fireworks.'
—(quoted in The End of Overeating by David A. Kessler)

The biggest reason so many of us are overweight and obese today is that we're surrounded by very convenient, highly processed, *hyperpalatable* foods.

You may not have come across the word *hyperpalatable*. Hyperpalatable is a word coined by David Kessler, the former commissioner of the Food and Drug Administration, in his book *The End of Overeating*. It's an extension of the word "palatable", which means pleasant tasting. So, hyperpalatable is a food that is *very* pleasant, that hits our "sweet spot" in terms of taste.

But it's not just taste. Hyperpalatable foods hit our sweet spot in terms of *everything*. Crunch, sweetness, creaminess, texture, even how many times we need to chew it before it goes down— hyperpalatable foods have been engineered to optimize *all* these.

***

Here's a thought experiment. Imagine that you have a bowl of plain white sugar in front of you, and a spoon. You're not really full, but you're also not really hungry. There's a glass of water available if you want it.

Do you want to eat spoonful after spoonful of sugar? Are you tempted; do you feel like you *must* have sugar?

I'm guessing the answer is *no*. The temptation just isn't there. Plain sugar is just not very attractive on its own. It doesn't appeal to us.

Here's another scenario. This one is the same, except for butter. You have a stick of plain butter on a plate in front of you, with a knife and fork for convenience.

Do you feel the urge to cut yourself a slice of butter and take a bite, and then another, and then another? Does it tempt you to eat more and more—to eat the whole thing?

I doubt it. I don't think you'll be tempted to overindulge in plain butter. You probably wouldn't even take a single bite. You weren't very tempted by the sugar, and butter is the same—it's just not tempting when it's just the one thing, alone.

But let's look at one last scenario. Suppose you have a package of Oreo cookies in front of you. It's your favorite variety—perhaps the Double Stuff or Thins.

Would you eat a few cookies? Might you even eat much of the package?

The situation now is *very* different. We're not talking about just sweet, or just fat, like we were with the sugar and the butter. We're talking about a highly engineered product, with the *exact* right combination of fat and sugar to tempt us.

***

The people who develop products like these have advanced degrees in chemistry, and have titles such as food chemist, molecular gastronomist, and flavor chemist. They've spent tens of thousands of hours on this particular product, and products like it. Entire careers are spent making highly processed food, like Oreos and foods like it, into a deliciously tempting, addictive eating experience.

Many people would eat the whole package of Oreos, or whatever hyperpalatable food was most tempting to them. A friend of mine had to stop buying Betty Crocker Rich and Creamy Frosting. She used it to frost the cupcakes she occasionally baked, but then found that her teenage daughter would eat whole cans, with a spoon, while binge-watching television.

These foods are so tempting, and go down so easily, that most people eat far more than what the package calls a "serving". Years ago, I would definitely have overindulged. This is before I realized the danger in these types of food.

✳✳✳

Let's go back to some of the stories of famine and hunger that I wrote about earlier. People then were in situations of real hunger, situations where they would die if they didn't find some food. Of course, they would have eaten the plain sugar, or plain butter. People in starvation situations ate all kinds of foods that we wouldn't even consider food, like grass and tree bark. That helped them survive.

However, we don't live like that today. There's plenty of food available, and we spend less money on food (as a percentage of income) than any other society in history. That's why these days, we probably wouldn't eat the plain sugar, or plain butter. We definitely wouldn't binge on it.

But we *would* eat the Oreo cookies. We might even binge on them.

If the Oreo cookies don't appeal to you, then perhaps fresh glazed Dunkin Donuts, or delectable Doritos corn chips? There's probably some combination of what is basically fat and sugar, or fat and salt, that is *deeply* appealing to you. It's likely that many foods would tempt you to overeat, far beyond the call of hunger.

These are the *hyperpalatable* foods. Foods that call to you, that you crave. Foods that are very difficult to resist

✻✻✻

Let's look more closely at what hyperpalatable foods are like. First of all, of course, we're not talking about simple foods with one ingredient. We're not talking about apples, plain rice, boiled eggs, bananas, or cooked chicken breast, or any foods like that.

Instead, these are just a few examples of hyperpalatable foods:

- Cheetos Crunchy Cheddar Jalapeno Cheese Flavored Snacks
- McDonald's Bacon Smokehouse burger
- T.G. I. Friday's Loaded Cheddar & Bacon Potato Skins
- Reese's Peanut Butter Puffs breakfast cereal
- CLIF BAR - Sweet & Salty Energy Bar - Peanut Butter & Honey with Sea Salt

These are not simple foods, ones that our ancestors have eaten for centuries. Hyperpalatable foods are complex. Many different ingredients are put together in combinations that delight our taste buds. They stimulate and excite us. Layers upon layers of flavor, of fat, sweet, and salt, combine to make them irresistible.

Another feature of the hyperpalatable foods is that they have a lot of calories, packed into a small volume. Six Oreo cookies are the equivalent of 3 bananas, in calories. But the bananas are much bulkier and heavier, with more water and fiber. Also, the bananas have no fat, while the Oreos have a lot.

This is called calorie density. The Oreos have a much higher calorie density, and our bodies crave dense, high-calorie foods. Most people could easily eat six Oreo cookies at a time. And for many

23

people, they wouldn't stop until the package was empty. But few people would eat three bananas at a time.

In the example of the T.G. I. Friday's Loaded Cheddar & Bacon Potato Skins, the potato is hollowed out, fried, then piled high with sour cream, cheese, and bacon. Or take buffalo chicken wings. The fattiest part of the chicken is pre-fried, shipped to the restaurant frozen, fried again, then glazed, and served with creamy and spicy dipping sauces. It usually comes with some celery sticks, to give the illusion that we're eating something healthy.

✱✱✱

So, we've looked at what hyperpalatable foods are like. But what could possibly be wrong with having easy access to delicious, abundant food? Food that delights us, food that makes eating fun? This is something humans have desired and fantasized about throughout all of history. What's wrong with it?

Here's the problem. Most people find it very difficult to avoid these foods when they're easily available. And it's also difficult for them to stop eating, once they've started. These foods are designed to be delicious, and convenient to eat. They're hard to resist.

Humans have lived throughout almost all of our history in a situation of scarcity and hunger. Our drive to eat and our eating behavior helped us survive.

But now, the situation is different. Today, we live in a food environment of extreme abundance. Food is everywhere. Most of it is hyperpalatable food—highly engineered food products designed to make us crave them.

In this situation, *most* people will gain weight. They will gain weight to the point that their health will suffer.

Can hyperpalatable foods be addictive?

There's been a lot of debate about hyperpalatable foods, and whether they can be called addictive. On the one hand—we need to eat food, otherwise we'll die of starvation. How could we call food addictive, then?

But on the other hand, research shows us that *some* foods cause people to have very strong reactions. These reactions include constantly thinking about the foods, and not being able to stop eating them. These reactions are similar to the behaviors that people have with addictive drugs. Brain scans done in MRI machines show these similarities as well. So do studies with rats, given these types of foods.

These are the hyperpalatable foods—foods that we find extremely delicious. They're highly processed, high-calorie, and engineered with just the right amounts of fat, sugar, and salt. They have just the perfect amount of crunch, and are easy and convenient to eat. They may not yet be technically defined as addictive, but all the evidence is pointing in that direction.

Think back to the crack cocaine epidemic of the 1980s. Crack cocaine is a refined form of cocaine, and is very addictive. It gives you a short but very intense high when smoked. Looking back at the history of this drug, we have:

- The original coca leaves—widely available in South America, chewed in the raw form (the actual leaf) for a

25

mild buzz. Archeological digs show that coca leaves have been used for at least 8000 years

- Cocaine—a processed form of coca leaves, first refined from the leaves in 1855. Cocaine is a commonly used addictive drug
- Crack cocaine—a more highly processed form of cocaine. Crack cocaine delivers a very fast high which leads to an even stronger addiction than cocaine.

This is how a drug evolves from a natural form, that gives you a mild buzz, to extremely addictive and appealing crack cocaine.

Hyperpalatable foods have taken a similar path. From basic foods, eaten for thousands of years, foods have become more and more highly processed. Food manufacturers and restaurants have gone through decades of experiments, and trial and error. They've discovered which types of processing and which combinations of ingredients appeal to us most. They've discovered which foods cause us to eat even when we're not hungry, and which foods make us come back for more, again and again.

Another component of the addictiveness of these foods is that they give instant pleasure. This is what's known in addiction research as "rapid reward". The hyperpalatable foods that people binge on are usually *not* dishes that they've slaved over in the kitchen. It's not the roast that has simmered on the stove the whole afternoon, or the special occasion cake that took hours to prepare.

No, the addictive foods are the instant pleasure foods, that require no work at all. Foods like ice cream, packaged snacks like cookies, chips, and candy, fast food—these are the most dangerous foods. The pleasure comes right away, and requires little work or preparation. It takes just seconds to rip open a package of chips and start enjoying it. Just like with addictive drugs—there's an immediate reward.

These foods may not yet be defined as "addictive". But they're very close, and we need to understand that most people are very vulnerable to them.

Portion Size

Have you ever been to a museum that had common household items from about a hundred years ago? I was at a local historical museum recently, and noticed the dinner plates and serving bowls. These plates and bowls were from around the 1920s.

They were remarkable, because they looked *so small*, compared to dinner plates and serving bowls today. The dinner plates back then were about the size of a salad plate or large dessert plate now. Serving bowls from the 1920s were about the same size as a larger soup bowl from today.

And of course, this increase in plate size reflects increases in how much we're eating. Many studies have shown that larger plates and bowls result in larger portion sizes, thus more calories.

Here are a few examples of portion size changes:

- When McDonald's started, in 1955, there was one size of french fries. It was smaller than the smallest french fries today.
- The size of an average bagel has more than doubled.
- The average serving of soda is almost three times the size it was in the 1950s.

- Orange juice fifty years ago was served in juice glasses, which were 4 to 6 ounces. Now, you'll get orange juice served to you in regular sized glasses, which will give you at least 12 ounces. That's double the juice, and double the calories.
- The cookie that you buy in a coffee shop is about five times the size of what used to be a normal size cookie.

We could go on and on with these examples. It's not that restaurant owners or food manufacturers want to make us fat—they don't, not specifically. They just want us to buy their products. Consumers show a preference for the "better value" with what they buy, and what they don't buy. What happens if the hamburgers at one restaurant are 50% larger than at another, but are otherwise similar and have similar prices? Most often, consumers will go to the restaurant that offers the "better deal"—the larger burger.

So, these changes in portion size are driven by consumer demand. They're driven by the desire to get a good value, to get more bang for the buck. It's a natural human tendency. For instance, say you're debating whether to buy something like a breakfast muffin. If it's larger than you expect, that may make you more likely to buy it. You feel you're getting a good deal. Restaurants that do *not* cater to our desire for a better value will go out of business.

What happens when the "standard" size serving of a common food increases? If the size of a bagel doubles, do we eat only half of the bagel, and take the rest home?

No. We eat the whole thing. When a standard serving gets larger, that *normalizes* the larger serving in our minds. The larger serving becomes the new standard.

If we were given what was previously a normal size bagel, it now looks like a mini-bagel—a serving for a child. We would feel short-changed.

Variety

Why is it that there's always room for dessert? Say you're at a restaurant, and have just filled up with a satisfying dinner of tasty spaghetti and meatball pasta, with some sides.

Then the waiter presents you with the dessert menu. And suddenly, you have some room. The different dessert options are described in mouth-watering detail, and some of them sound very appetizing. You really want to enjoy one. But just moments before, you were completely full. How can this be?

The scientific term for this is "sensory-specific satiety". You're tired of the rich, meaty tastes that you enjoyed earlier. They don't appeal to you anymore. But now a whole new flavor of foods is presented to you—sweets. And it's appealing again. You feel a strong desire to eat. This is how variety encourages us to overeat.

Throughout human history, this would have been a very useful behavior to have. Mostly, our ancestors didn't stick to one food, or limited foods. When possible, our ancestors ate a variety of different foods when they were available. This habit helped them get all the nutrition they needed.

But now, the amount of food variety that surrounds us has exploded. And this is not a variety of different fruits and vegetables. Instead, it's a variety of highly processed, hyperpalatable foods.

Constantly being surrounded by this kind of variety is a huge contributor to overeating, and therefore obesity. As recently as the 1990s, supermarkets contained about 7,000 items. Currently, the average supermarket contains 50,000 items. Most of these are highly processed, hyperpalatable foods, designed to be convenient and addictive.

***

Rats are much easier to study than humans. You just put them in a cage, and feed them whatever you want. The studies that would be unethical to do on humans, we can do on rats. And there are multiple rat studies showing that *variety causes overeating*. The more variety, the more we eat.

Rats that are just given "rat chow"—standard rat food, with complete nutrition but not particularly exciting—eat much less than those offered more variety. Rats that are offered strawberry milkshakes, as well as chocolate milkshakes eat much more than rats whose only food is rat chow. Rats that are given these two milkshake flavors *at the same meal* eat much more than those that are offered strawberry flavor one day, and chocolate flavor the next.

Humans behave the same as rats, when it comes to food variety. When offered a *variety* of tasty food choices, we eat much more than when we're just offered one tasty food.

It's the buffet effect, and I'm sure you're familiar with it. If you're at a buffet, with a large selection of delicious food, you'll eat much more than if you were just offered one food—even your favorite.

Again, throughout almost all of human history, this would have been a good thing. If you ate more, you would be able to survive famines and periods of hunger. But in today's world, this urge to enjoy as much variety as we can is not serving us well. It's one of the factors causing us to gain unhealthy amounts of weight.

Many years ago, it was rare to have a large variety of foods available—it happened only on holidays or special occasions. Now, variety and abundance surround us, to the point that every day could be a special occasion. It's no surprise that we weigh more than ever before.

Cultural changes

The culture surrounding food has changed in the past 100 years, in the past 50 years, and even in the past 20 years. Before, eating was an event that required preparation. It happened with other people. Food was eaten on named occasions—breakfast, lunch, or dinner—or special social occasions. Snacks were rare.

Compare that to now. Eating takes place everywhere. Every occasion, even ones that weren't linked with food before, is an eating occasion. And snacking is acceptable at any time, and everywhere. It's never rude to eat in front of people, to eat on the bus, to eat while walking down the street.

In some countries, like Japan (with an extremely low 3% obesity rate), it is still rude to eat casually in front of other people. But not in the United States. In the United States, it's accepted and promoted.

Snacking opportunities surround us. Vending machines selling chips or candy bars are in most workplaces and schools. A casual stroll at the mall tempts you with the smell of sweet cinnamon rolls (the Cinnabon Classic Roll has a mind-boggling 880 calories). Many social and cultural changes occurred in the 1980s, which is when obesity really started skyrocketing. One of these changes is that people started eating fewer meals together, and began snacking much more. Some researchers claim that *most* of the extra calories that we're consuming these days come from snacks.

These cultural changes around food and eating have been like a tsunami. Traditions and social norms about eating have been swept away. Below are just a few of the many examples of situations and events that have become eating occasions in today's society.

✳✳✳

Organized kids' soccer used to be a place where actually playing soccer was the highlight. But now, for many kids, the after-game snack is the main event. I've been to soccer games where parents brought 4 items for each kid—bottles of Gatorade in all the colors of the rainbow, peel-off "fruit" candy, bags of Goldfish crackers, and maybe a stick of mozzarella cheese as a token "healthy food".

✳✳✳

A schoolteacher friend described the Valentine's Day extravaganza that her school's Parent Teacher Association put on. There were bowls of different heart-shaped candies and chocolates, and all kinds of Valentine's Day themed red, pink, and white snacks.
Another friend, also a teacher, described her school's lavish teacher appreciation week. Every day of that week, the teachers received treats and goodies from the Parent Teacher Association. For instance, a "cookie blizzard", a catered breakfast, etc.

32

✳✳✳

A former boss of mine would always bring in multiple boxes of doughnuts for his team every Wednesday. People looked forward to "Doughnut Wednesday". Another former boss would always bring a treat for regular meetings. She brought in two dozen assorted bagels and a variety of different spreadable cream cheeses– plain, salmon, honey, and chives.

Restaurants

Another huge cultural change that's happened recently is eating out. Years ago, most people rarely went out to eat. And many never ate out at all. When I was growing up in the 1970s and 80s, my family rarely ate in a restaurant. And we were typical of most middle-class families of that time.

That's changed, and very dramatically. Here's a quote from a 1956 ad in a popular magazine, sponsored by a restaurant association:

Eating out gives life a lift! When you take your family out to eat, it's all fun, no fuss, and a delightful change. Mother has a holiday from kitchen duties...Dad is thanked for his thoughtfulness...youngsters love it!

These days, we don't need to be reminded to eat in restaurants. Eating in restaurants—fancy, mid-range, and fast food—is something that most families do often, even multiple times a week. Restaurant eating goes hand-in-hand with the decline of home cooking. And when eating in restaurants, people tend to eat many

33

more calories than when they eat at home. The portion sizes, continuously being tempted with extras (drinks, appetizers, desserts, etc.), all of these contribute to extra calories. Further on in the book, I'll go into more details on the specifics of how restaurants promote overeating (short answer: they're just helping us do what we want to do anyway), but for now, be aware that restaurants are a big factor in our collective weight gain.

∗∗∗

Changes in our culture and society are causing people to become overweight. And it's a circular process—as more people become overweight, the more accepted and common it is. It becomes easier and easier to eat in a way that causes weight gain. It becomes harder and harder to eat more traditionally—the way people ate 100 years ago, before the majority of us became overweight.

Here's how that works. Take a statistically average woman in the United States today, who is overweight, with a body mass index of 29. A body mass index of 29 puts her at the very top of the overweight category, and almost in the obese category.

About 100 years ago, this same woman would have been noticeable, walking down the street. She would have looked different from everyone else, because very few people were around her weight. There was not a huge variety of convenient, highly processed, addictive food around. There would have been no ready-made clothing available in her size, so all her clothing would have been custom-made, at great expense.

But today, this same woman doesn't look outside of the norm at all. She looks about average, because she is average, statistically.

"Average" has changed completely. Since most other people are heavier as well, she doesn't stand out. She sees lots of people that are approximately her weight. The foods that cause obesity—highly processed, hyperpalatable convenience foods—surround her and everyone else most of the time. There's plenty of clothing available in her size, no need to go to plus-size stores. So, the pressure to lose weight is much less.

The problem with abundance

Prosperity is a wonderful thing. The fact that famine has disappeared in much of the world is an amazing achievement.

But there's also a flip side to this achievement. It's because of our prosperity, and the changes in our culture that have come along with it, that the *majority* of Americans are now overweight or obese. And the majority of Americans are suffering from the discomfort, and potential disease and disability, that go along with being overweight or obese.

Think of that. The vast majority of Americans are now overweight or obese. More than 71% of people in the United States are overweight or obese now, and in some groups it's much higher.

Here's what some people without weight issues say:

Well, nobody is putting the food in your mouth. Nobody is making you chew and swallow. Just stop eating so much junk!

I've seen this type of comment a lot. I'm sure you have as well. But if the vast majority of people have issues with overeating—is it really a willpower issue? Is the problem *really* that overweight people just have no self-control?

No. It's our food environment that has changed. It's changed dramatically, to the point that it's a completely different world. This has extreme consequences for our weight. It's a problem of constant temptation by highly desirable, hyperpalatable foods.

One of the most difficult things to do is to have delicious, tempting snacks and treats available, right in front of you, where you can see and smell them, *and not eat them.* If they're crunchy foods like potato chips, perhaps you can even hear other people eating them. All of your senses are being stimulated by these foods.

***

It's not easy or straightforward to do studies on humans. But in many aspects of our biology, humans are very similar to rats. And studies on lab rats have conclusively shown that the *only* thing a rat needs to become obese is to have delicious, tempting food constantly available.

This fact was first discovered by Anthony Sclafani. Sclafani was a graduate student in the late 1960s, researching the causes of overeating. He was trying to get rats to become obese, and was having a very difficult time. Sclafani tried giving the rats as much rat chow as they wanted. He switched out the regular rat chow for high-fat rat chow. But no luck—the rats didn't gain much weight.

Then he switched his strategy. Instead of giving the rats standard rat chow, he gave them a variety of tempting foods. He offered the rats a constant, all-you-can-eat buffet of foods like chocolate-chip cookies, salami, chocolate, marshmallows, and sugary Froot Loops breakfast cereal. And that's all it took. The rats quickly became obese, doubling their weight compared to the control rats.

This experiment is one that has been done many times, and always gives the same results. If rats are constantly surrounded by these types of foods, they gain massive amounts of weight. Rats are similar to humans when it comes to appetite and eating, and when this type of experiment has been done with humans, the results have been the same. Being surrounded by a variety of abundant, delicious foods is all it takes for most people to gain weight.

So, we don't need to come up with complicated theories about why we're gaining weight. It's not about too much fat, or too many carbs. It's not that we're suffering from more emotional trauma now, compared to 100 years ago.

Human beings—and rats—don't have it in their nature to constantly say "no" when they're surrounded by delicious foods. All it takes to gain weight is to live in a food environment of constant temptation. This is exactly what we have today. And that's why so many of us are overweight and obese.

✳✳✳

Let's talk about blame, and responsibility. It's unkind and not useful to blame people who are overweight or obese for their weight problem. And it just doesn't work for people with a weight problem to blame or shame themselves.

But what about responsibility? Responsibility is a completely different thing. Responsibility is not about blaming yourself—it's about recognizing reality. It's about understanding that there's only one person who can make a change for yourself, and that's *you*.

You are the one who can learn:

- The history of hunger, and how it created our strong urge to eat
- How vulnerable we can be to certain foods
- Why our current food environment is so tempting, and so unhealthy

And you're the one that can figure out:

- How weighing yourself daily can help you fight our unhealthy food environment
- What habits are causing your weight gain
- The food rules and guidelines you could use to lose weight, and keep it off

Responsibility. You are the only one with the *ability* to *respond* to an unhealthy, addictive food environment. There's nobody else.

Why am I spending so much time on the history of obesity, and our current food environment? Why is it important to understand these topics?

Here's why. Once you realize that the *main* reason for the explosion in obesity is because we're now almost constantly surrounded by tempting foods, then you have a huge advantage in losing weight. You have two weapons in your mental toolbox, for reaching a healthy weight and staying there. Here are these weapons:

- **You understand that blaming yourself or feeling ashamed of your weight is useless**. The majority of people—more than 71 percent—in the United States are overweight or obese now. Instead of shame or blame, save your energy. You'll need it for figuring out strategies and tactics that work *for you.*

- **You realize that you must fight your food environment**. It's because of our unhealthy food environment that we're gaining so much weight. So, you need to figure out how to fight your food environment. We'll talk about the details later, but understanding the enemy is half the battle.

What about genetics? Isn't weight gain partly about genetics, too? Don't some people have more of a tendency to be overweight because of their genes?

It's true. Some people do have a stronger tendency to gain weight, because they have a stronger drive to eat. Suppose that your parents or grandparents were obese back in the 1970s or earlier. Remember that back then, the rate of obesity was much, much lower. If that's your situation, then what does this mean for you?

It may mean that hyperpalatable foods are even *more* tempting for you than for most people. This doesn't mean you can't lose weight— not at all. But it does mean that limiting your choices might be even more important for you than for other people. Later in this book, I talk about personal food rules. These are rules you make for yourself, to limit temptation, and avoid the need to constantly decide what to eat. If you have a family history of obesity, then you'll want to give particular attention to food rules.

But because human history includes so much famine and hunger, *everybody* has a strong drive to eat. For some people it's stronger than average. This doesn't change the fact that the *majority* of people in the United States are now overweight or obese. A hundred years ago, the number was only a tiny fraction of what it is today. Have our genes changed so much in these past 100 years, that we can blame our weight gain on genetics?

Of course not. Our genes can't change that quickly. Our weight gain is caused by our food environment. It's caused by the fact that hyperpalatable food—food that is extremely tempting and appealing—is relatively cheap and almost always around.

We're now in a situation that humanity has wished for throughout history. We're surrounded by delicious, abundant food. But the old saying, "Be careful what you wish for" definitely applies here. Because when it gets to the point it's at now, abundance becomes a problem. It leads directly to severe problems with obesity.

Summary

- Losing weight and keeping it off gets much easier when you understand why people have gained so much weight in the last 50 or so years. You need to understand the cause of the problem in order to solve it.
- In the past 50 years, people have gained a tremendous amount of weight. Now, more than 71 percent of adults in the US are overweight or obese.
- Human history is full of times of severe hunger and famine. To survive, our ancestors developed a very strong drive to eat high-calorie food when it was around. We inherited this drive from our ancestors.
- Today, our food environment includes:
  - Extreme abundance

- o More variety in foods than people have ever had before
- o Mostly convenience foods—just open the package and start eating
- o Hyperpalatable foods, designed to be addictive
- Our weight gain is caused by a mismatch between our strong biological urge to eat whenever delicious food is available—and the fact that today, this food is always available.
- Blaming and shaming yourself is useless. Save your energy to figure out how to overcome the food environment we live in.

WHY WEIGHING YOURSELF DAILY IS ESSENTIAL

How the habit of stepping on the scale every morning can help you lose weight

---

You probably picked up this book because you're hoping to lose weight, and want to get some more information on how to best do that. In this chapter, I hope to convince you of one thing:

A rock-solid habit of weighing yourself, every single day, is fundamental to weight loss and—especially—keeping the weight off.

The evidence that this is true has been building for the last decade. More and more studies are coming out, showing that a daily weigh-in is strongly linked to weight loss.

This is not a quick fix. This is a process of getting used to stepping on the scale every day, and checking your weight. And it's not magic—you still need to reflect and work on the food habits that are affecting your weight.

But for many years, people have been explicitly told that they should *not* weigh themselves daily. They've been told they're too fragile, that it would damage them emotionally.

I'd like to persuade you that the *opposite* is true.

Being overweight or obese causes significant health issues, and often causes emotional problems as well. The best single habit you can develop to get to a healthy weight, and stay there, is to weigh yourself.

Every single day.

The psychology of a daily weigh-in— why it works

The first principle is that you must not fool yourself—and you are the easiest person to fool.
—Richard Feynman

Why would weighing yourself daily, and logging it, be so helpful when you're trying to lose weight, or maintain your weight? The reasons it works aren't necessarily obvious.

A big reason why it's so helpful is that monitoring *anything* leads to awareness. And awareness is the first step of change. For many people, merely stepping on the scale and writing down their weight can lead to weight loss. One study was done comparing two groups

44

of overweight people, both given some very basic weight loss advice. The target group was asked to weigh themselves daily, and the control group was not.

Which group lost a significant amount of weight? As you'd expect, the one that weighed themselves daily lost weight, and the control group did not.

How is this possible? The group weighing themselves daily had not signed up for a new diet program. They weren't receiving packaged meals as part of the study. They didn't have a weight counselor, and weren't getting any additional advice or tips on weight loss.

And yet they lost weight. And the group that was *not* weighing themselves daily did not.

***

What's happening is not magic, it's *measuring*. Stepping on the scale, noting the number, and writing it down. All these things, combined, caused the study group members to make different choices throughout their day.

These could have been simple things—maybe choosing half a bagel instead of a whole. Or drinking black coffee instead of drinking a sugary latte. But these choices combined to slowly, gradually reduce their weight.

Stepping on the scale, and writing down the number on the scale every morning gave them a push to make healthier decisions during the day. It did *not* increase their willpower. It just balanced out their decision-making.

Let me explain. Throughout the day, we're faced with many, many food decisions. For instance, suppose you work in an office, and it's your coworker's birthday. A huge tray of enormous cupcakes has been brought in from the new gourmet bakery down the street. Everyone's been talking about this new place, and how delicious their cupcakes are.

Here's what the factors in your decision would look like, if you hadn't weighed yourself that morning.

Without a daily weigh-in habit

Eat the cupcake

- These cupcakes smell delicious
- Everyone's having some
- I deserve a treat

Don't eat the cupcake

- I don't need it
- It's unhealthy
- I'll gain weight if I eat this type of food

And here's what it would look like, if you had just weighed yourself that morning, and knew you would weigh yourself again the next morning:

With a daily weigh-in habit

Eat the cupcake

- These cupcakes smell delicious
- Everyone's having some
- I deserve a treat

Don't eat the cupcake

- I don't need it
- It's unhealthy
- I'll gain weight if I eat this type of food
- *My weight this morning was down a little, I want to keep that going*

You'll notice that there's another factor, when you have a daily weigh-in habit:

My weight this morning was down a little, I want to keep that going

That additional reason—your weight this morning and knowing that you'll weigh yourself again tomorrow—can be a huge help when you're faced with a choice. You've added another piece of information to the thoughts and feelings bouncing around in your head. It's recent—from this morning. It's recorded—you physically wrote down your weight a few hours ago.

If the number on your scale had been up that morning, your self-talk would have been different. It might have been something like "I've been mostly doing fine with my weight, but it was up yesterday. I don't want it to be up two days in a row".

But either way, it would have given you a nudge towards making a healthier decision. It would have made the cupcake less tempting. You're surrounded—like we all are—by a food environment that overwhelms us with the sights and smells of delicious foods. If we eat these foods without limits, we'll become overweight, or regain lost weight. Your daily weigh-in will give you a daily boost of motivation, and will remind you how your weight is trending. And just *having* that information, from that very morning, will help you make better decisions.

Why your scale seems wrong sometimes

I've been weighing myself daily for many years. And I can tell you from experience that the scale really is your honest, blunt friend. Your weight in the morning is, mostly, a decent indicator of how you ate yesterday. That's why it's so helpful—it's almost immediate feedback. It takes only seconds to step on the scale. And you can't fool yourself, like you can when you're counting calories.

Even though your morning weigh-in on the scale is *usually* a good reflection on what you ate yesterday, there are a few reasons the number may surprise you. Sometimes, you can have a perfectly healthy day, in terms of what you ate and drank. You ate reasonable meals. You didn't overindulge. And yet the scale is up.

Here are some reasons why this happens:

You ate more carbohydrates than normal

Carbohydrates (bread, rice, oatmeal, etc.) are a good source of glycogen, which is a body chemical that's used as a fuel. And one interesting feature of glycogen is that 1 gram of glycogen will bond to 3 or 4 grams of water.

What does this mean in practical terms? If you've had a day when you've eaten more carbohydrates than you normally do, your weight may be up because of water retention. This could be the case even if you don't eat more total calories than normal.

That's why there's often a substantial weight loss at the very beginning of a low-carb diet. The body's stores of glycogen are lower, and all the water associated with it is less.

You ate more salty foods than normal

Another reason that your weight may be higher than you expect is that you've eaten more salt than you normally do. It could be that you just ate a bag of chips. Or you're eating more processed foods, which are high in salt. And since eating more salt causes you to crave and drink more water, that alone can cause water retention. And that extra water will stay until the extra salt is flushed out of your body.

Constipation

Not having a bowel movement for a few days will affect your weight. You can become more regular by eating more fiber, especially natural fiber in foods such as vegetables, fruits, and whole grains.

Sometimes our bowel movements are not regular, even if we eat plenty of fiber. This happens especially as we get older, or when we're traveling. If this is the case, then weighing yourself daily is even more important, because you will get a better sense for what your normal weight range is.

You scale isn't accurate

I was reviewing some online weight loss forums, and saw this:

The next morning, I stepped on the scale again. This time it read 181 pounds. That means I lost 10 pounds in one day. That can't be correct.

If you truly lost 10 pounds in one day, you're doing something strange and unhealthy. What this really means is that your scale isn't accurate, and you should buy another one, right away.

Purchase a new digital bathroom scale, with good reviews. Take a look at the section entitled "What kind of scale should I buy" for more on this topic.

Don't let worries about scale accuracy get you off track. Modern digital bathroom scales are very accurate.

You're weighing yourself at different times during the day

You should always weigh yourself in the morning, just after going to the bathroom and before breakfast. That's your most consistent weight. If you weigh yourself later on in the day, you'll get more random variations from all kinds of factors—the meal you just ate, the two cups of coffee you had, etc.

...You just ate too much

There are a few other reasons that your weight can be higher than you expected. For instance, women sometimes retain water just before their period. And intense exercise can cause inflammation, which may cause you to retain water.

If you're weighing yourself daily, you'll get a good sense for these minor ups and downs in your weight, and they won't bother you. You'll probably be able to predict what your weight will be.

But here's the thing: if your weight is higher than you expect, over more than a few days or a week, it's almost certainly *not* because of any of the above.

The most likely cause is that you ate too much. Maybe you're misjudging food quantities. Or the regular drink you order at the coffee shop just has too many calories, and is more like a milkshake than coffee. Perhaps the sandwich you had for lunch yesterday had more calories than you thought—maybe you should have ordered a half-sandwich instead of a whole sandwich.

This is exactly why weighing yourself daily is such a critical health habit, both for losing weight and maintaining a steady weight. The scale is your honest, blunt friend. Sure, there will be weight gains that are caused by factors like eating salty foods, or extra carbs, or when you last had a bowel movement.

But many of your gains—and all the weight gains that stay there, day after day—are caused by just plain eating and drinking too much. And these eating and drinking choices are habits that you can change.

Seeing the number on the scale will help you in many ways. It will:

- *Motivate* you to make changes
- *Give you feedback* on which habit changes help you lose weight, and which don't
- *Warn you* of the gradual weight gain that happens with so many of us, over the years

People sometimes say "Ignorance is bliss". That may be true sometimes. But when it comes to getting to a healthy weight, and staying there, this saying works much better:

Knowledge Is Power

Why not just weigh yourself weekly?

Weight loss programs and counselors often recommend weighing yourself weekly. This recommendation is slowly changing as the evidence piles up, showing the benefit of daily weighing. But it's a very gradual process.

Here are some of the reasons that weighing yourself daily is a much better choice than weekly.

It's easier to remember daily instead of weekly.

Things that you do daily are much easier to remember than things you need to do only once a week. When you're weighing yourself every day, you just put the scale right next to the shower, and weigh yourself just before you step in the shower. Or choose whichever point in your morning routine that's easiest for you.

The point is that by doing something daily instead of weekly, there's no thinking involved. You don't need to remember if it's the correct day of the week for weighing yourself. The less you have to think about it, the more likely it is to get done.

Do you have any weekly habits, that you do without a reminder? Most people don't. For me, I need to remember to take the garbage out to the street once a week on Tuesday. And I need a reminder in my calendar to do this, every Tuesday evening, otherwise I'll forget.

But daily habits are different. People often have many daily habits that are rock-solid. And they're usually morning habits, too, which is perfect because that's when you should weigh yourself. These are habits like brushing your teeth, taking a shower, etc.

Because of that, it's easy to hook a daily weigh-in habit into your daily routine. For instance, you may want to put the scale right next to the shower, to remind you to weigh in before you shower.

Weekly habits, though? There's not usually much to hook it onto, there's nothing to "trigger" it. It's harder to make it work, without tedious reminders.

Weekly habits are more likely to disappear than daily habits

Weighing yourself *weekly* can very easily slip into weighing yourself *never*. Suppose Rachel plans to weigh herself every Sunday. Then Monday comes, and she remembers that she missed her weigh-in on Sunday. She thinks, "Oops, didn't do it yesterday, I'll weigh myself next Sunday". But then a few events come up during the week, like heavy restaurant meals, a birthday, etc. She knows that her weight will be up. She's a little worried about it. And that leads Rachel to avoid weighing herself next Sunday.

It's a slippery slope. And avoiding the scale leads to anxiety about stepping on it—an anxiety that wouldn't exist if you stepped on the scale every single day.

This is how many people gain weight. It's not because they're weighing themselves every day, and saying "Darn, I gained half a pound". No, they stop weighing entirely, because it's uncomfortable. This can last for years, and cause massive weight gain.

Daily weigh-ins provide daily feedback—feedback you need to make healthier choices

When you weigh-in weekly, it's seen as a "moment of truth". But that's the *last* thing your weight should be.

It's not a moment of truth. It's a number that can help you check how you ate and drank over the last few days. You might decide, based on the number, if you need to re-evaluate your food habits. Maybe you splurged yesterday on a special meal, and your weight shows this. You may choose to eat more lightly today.

If you're weighing daily, the number on the scale will remind you of what went well, and what didn't. You'll think—hey, I had a huge lunch yesterday, I'm definitely bringing a light lunch today. The number will *help* you.

What if you're weighing in just once a week? You've probably eaten 21 meals, and lots of snacks. Are you going to remember them all? No. And since you won't remember them, there's no way you'll be able to figure which habits you need to adjust, or which choices you could improve.

And improving your habits and choices is the key to managing your weight.

Weekly weigh-ins cause more anxiety than daily weigh-ins

There are many commercial weight loss companies that promote weekly weigh-ins, at their centers. The weigh-ins, and the "accountability" that they provide, are part of what you're paying for when you sign up.

But what happens when you only weigh-in weekly? The main thing is that your weight will be a surprise. It may be a pleasant surprise; it may be an unpleasant surprise. But it can cause anxiety. Here's a quote from the website of one of these weight loss companies:

> *...it's that one tiny minute on the scale that seems to overshadow everything else. In that one minute, you're taken back to sitting in the class of the meanest teacher in school, waiting to get your math quiz back. Will you get an A? An F? And will it be the grade you deserve?*

Is this something you want to do? Does it sound like a healthy habit—one that you're motivated to keep up for a lifetime?

Of course not. This type of weigh-in is used for punishment or reward. It gives far too much importance to your weight. Stepping on the scale is a cause of anxiety instead of a useful daily tool.

Another common result of weekly weigh-ins is that you may feel devastated if your weight hasn't gone down. You think you've done well on eating habits during the week, so you weight *should* be down, at least a little.

But then you find you haven't lost any weight! And that's often the way the diet ends. Disappointment with the number at the weekly weigh-in causes discouragement. That discouragement leads to a full stop.

If you were weighing yourself daily, you wouldn't have that problem. There would be no surprise. The daily weigh-in gives you the nudge you need every day, to remind you to eat a little better or a little less. And those habits, carried out every day, will cause you to lose weight and not regain it.

Here's another quote, from the same weight loss company:

No wonder, then, that people put so much thought into coming up with the perfect weight-tracking-day strategy. What day? What time? What to wear?

This is wasted effort. If you're getting stressed out about trivial weigh-in details like what day, what time, and what to wear, then you're worrying about the wrong things. And you'll have less time and energy to put into what matters—adjusting your eating habits.

Weight fluctuations cause more problems if you're weighing yourself weekly

When I say weight fluctuations, I mean those changes in your weight that seem random. These are changes caused by things like water retention, not having had a bowel movement in a few days, etc. I'm *not* talking about weight changes that are caused by eating too much.

Here's what some people say:

Weigh yourself once a week, after you wake up every Monday morning. This eliminates things like water retention and bowel movements, which can cause changes in your weight.

But how could weighing yourself once a week, instead of once a day, eliminate fluctuations in weight? Do the random fluctuations somehow disappear on the one day of the week that you weigh yourself?

No, they don't disappear. The meaningless fluctuations are still there. In statistics, these fluctuations are sometimes called "noise." I discussed them in the section "Why your scale seems wrong sometimes." They're what we want to ignore. The real data—weight changes caused by fat loss—is what we'd like to track, but the noise can be confusing.

The mistake that some people make is thinking that taking fewer measurements—weighing yourself once a week instead of daily— means that there is less noise. But that's not what happens. There's the same amount of noise, but since you have fewer measurements, *it's harder to see real changes*.

With 7 numbers, you have a good idea of how your weight has gone up and down over a week. But if you have just one number, you have no sense of what normal ups and downs look like. And what if you happen to weigh yourself on a day when your weight is higher? You're more likely to get discouraged. If you have the numbers for every day of the week, to balance things out, it'll be easier to see the overall trend.

Here's another example. What if you wanted to get the average temperature for July? Would it be more accurate to take the temperature reading every single day in that month? Or would it be more accurate to measure it once a week?

Of course, you'll get a much more accurate number if you measure the temperature every day. If you only did it once a week, you could easily hit a few hotter days, and be far off from the true average.

"Moment of Truth" thinking and the problems it causes

Weighing yourself every day should be a part of your routine, a lifetime habit that is the foundation of both losing weight, and maintaining a healthy weight.

Unfortunately, many people believe the exact opposite of this. They believe that weighing yourself is the "Moment of Truth". They believe that it determines your value as a person, or whether you've been "good" or "bad".

Or they believe it's something you need to prepare yourself for, and gather up your courage to do. They may think that stepping on the scale, and learning your weight, is an "event". Perhaps they believe that weighing yourself can be traumatic.

The truth is, weighing yourself daily can be routine, easy, and stress-free. It is one of the most helpful tools you have for losing weight. And having that weigh-in habit makes the most important part of weight management—not gaining the weight back—much, much easier.

If you suffer from "Moment of Truth" thinking, you will need to work at developing the right attitude. But once you get used to it, weighing yourself can be something that you do in less than five seconds every morning. It'll be a routine that you don't even need to think about.

***

One of the reasons that "Moment of Truth" thinking is popular is because of shows like The Biggest Loser. The Biggest Loser is one of the most popular reality TV shows of the past few decades. The format of the show is simple. About a dozen contestants are chosen, all of them severely obese. The contestants are isolated at a remote location, and allowed almost no contact with family or friends. They spend their days doing hours and hours of intense exercise, and completing various challenges. The challenges may include being tempted with high-calorie foods, doing mini-marathons, competing with each other to determine who will be voted out, etc. The person who loses the most weight, as a percentage of initial body weight, wins a quarter of a million dollars.

A big component of the show is the very emotional "reveal" every week, where the contestants get weighed. This is the "Moment of Truth". The person who lost the least weight will be eliminated from the contest, and have to go back home. However, the contestant who lost the most may win extra prizes.

Everything is done to heighten the intensity, and make it an emotional, teary moment. It's full of suspense, and very interesting for the viewers. But how is it for the contestants?

Well, most of them lose tremendous amounts of weight very quickly. But, as I'm sure you've guessed, almost all the contestants gain the weight back. They gain it back, and more.

It would be almost impossible to keep the weight off, considering how they lost it. Not one single component of their weight loss was a permanent lifestyle change. For instance:

- Contestants were away from their home and daily routine.
- They were allowed to eat only the foods prepared for them
- They worked out for hours and hours every day, doing exercises they were told to do
- Stepping on the scale was a "Moment of Truth" event. Depending on what the scale said, they were either punished or rewarded.

How could somebody possibly *not* regain all their weight back, if this is how they lost it?

The worst part of the show was that it contributed to the idea that weighing yourself is an emotional event. The producers of the show wanted you to believe that stepping on the scale needs to be a big surprise, and something full of anxiety and drama.

That's great for the show—they want to make it sensational and interesting. But it's terrible for long term weight loss.

***

I hope that as you're reading this book, I'm convincing you that stepping on the scale every morning should be a part of your daily routine. It's should be as solid a part of your morning routine as showering in the morning, combing your hair, brushing your teeth, or making your bed. Whatever rock-solid morning habit that you have—your morning weigh-in should be right next to it. There should be no drama, and almost no surprise.

Below is a comment from Hannah on an online weight-loss forum, on her diet progress:

> *For a few weeks now, I've been working hard at eating well, and exercising. I changed my diet, and didn't eat junk food. Finally, I stepped on the scale. I was sure I would have lost weight. But the number was up instead of down. How could that possibly be? I was so discouraged. And I quit my diet.*

What *could* have happened in Hannah's story, if she had set up a scale, and taken a few seconds to weigh herself and log her weight daily? She probably would have had a day or two that were discouraging because of random fluctuations. And maybe there would have been a few days where she knew that the fluctuations were not random, that she ate too much the day before. She may have realized that there was a particular habit she needed to work on. Maybe something like bringing a healthier lunch from home, instead of eating out.

When you don't weigh yourself every day, you may think you're giving your weight *less* importance. But what happens is that it takes on even *more* importance, because of the element of mystery and

60

surprise. It can become a potentially discouraging "Moment of Truth".

If Hannah had weighed herself every day, she would have had:

- Useful information on how her daily food habits were going
- No surprise
- No "Moment of Truth"

And most importantly, there would have been *no reason to stop*. It would have been much easier for Hannah to keep on going, keep on working on her daily habits, her food environment, and her eating strategy.

Stepping on your scale daily is like looking at the speedometer when you're driving. You glance at it regularly. The sooner that you know you're going too fast, the better. Why? Because then you adjust your speed. You don't get anxious about it, but you also don't ignore it.

What are some myths about weighing yourself daily?

There are many companies, organizations, and individual weight loss counselors that will tell you, specifically, *not* to weigh yourself daily. This is slowly changing, as the evidence is steadily building in favor of weighing yourself daily. But the outdated "weekly weigh-in at most" recommendation still has a lot of momentum behind it.

Some of the companies telling you not to weigh yourself daily are doing it because it doesn't fit their business plan. For instance, if you searched online recently for "weighing yourself daily", the first result was an article with the title "5 Reasons to Stop Weighing Yourself Everyday".

I took a careful look at this company that posted this article. It turns out that their main product is an extremely expensive body composition analysis device. These machines tell you what your weight is, but that's not all. They give you all kinds of other information, such as your skeletal mass, water weight, body fat percentage, etc. It's very high tech. And it's so expensive that only large commercial weight loss centers can afford to buy this machine.

So, *of course*, they don't want people to believe that they can just use a cheap, convenient bathroom scale at home every day. If people believed that, there would be no need for their product.

✳✳✳

It's important to understand *why* people promote certain products and policies. For instance—would you count on a hairdresser to give you unbiased advice on how often you should have your hair cut?

No, of course not. A hairdresser would happily cut your hair every other week. She wants people to come in for frequent haircuts because she earns more money that way. She could probably come up with some great reasons why frequent haircuts would be a good idea.

It's just the same with the company I mentioned above, which makes the expensive body composition device. They really want you to believe that weighing yourself daily at home is *not* a good tool for weight loss. So, they write a very persuasive article called "5 Reasons to Stop Weighing Yourself Daily", and manage to get it to #1 in the search rankings.

Go ahead and take a look at the article if you want. But all the reasons they give are covered in the section "Why your scale seems wrong sometimes." They're just the completely normal and predictable reasons why the number on your scale can fluctuate—but twisted, to seem like reasons you should avoid your scale.

Here are a few of the most well-known myths about weighing yourself every day.

Myth: The reminder of your weight every morning will shake your confidence, and make you more likely to slip up.

Reality: The weight on your scale is a piece of information about your body. It's like your blood pressure, or your age. If your blood pressure is too high, you need to do something about it. If your weight is causing health issues, you try to lose weight. It's something that you can and should take ownership of. Stepping on the scale in the morning is a tool to help you, that same day, make better food choices. It will remind you to develop better food habits.

Over the short term, it's more comfortable to *not* step on the scale. There's the old saying, "ignorance is bliss". Not to mention "out of sight, out of mind" and "what you don't know can't hurt you".

Over the short term—the *very* short term—ignorance is comfortable. But the long term comes quicker than we think. And the long-term effects of ignoring weight gain are very serious.

Myth: Instead of weighing yourself daily, you should ask yourself: "How do I look in the mirror? Do I feel healthy? Do my clothes fit well?

Reality: Why would you want to trade one straightforward number (your weight), for some very subjective, vague, questions? Are you really going to decide, every morning, if you feel healthy, or if your clothes fit well? Will you assign a number to "How do you look in the mirror?"

These questions are impossible and impractical. What this is really saying is, "Don't weigh yourself. You might feel uncomfortable if you weigh yourself".

It's true, weighing yourself daily might feel uncomfortable at the beginning. If it's a new habit for you, it will take courage to step on the scale daily. It will take practice to start looking at your daily weigh-in as a useful, honest tool. But as you do it daily, and as you commit yourself to making it a lifetime habit, you will realize that it's the easiest, most practical tool that you have.

What really helps with motivation, and with keeping yourself on track, is seeing the small changes. Being able to measure and notice them, even if they're small, will keep you on the right track.

The people that encourage you to not weigh yourself—they're saying what many people want to hear. But the truth is that if you avoid the scale, you're avoiding the simplest, most straightforward tool you have. You're losing the one measurement that will be completely honest with you.

Myth: If you can't eliminate the emotional element attached to the number on the bathroom scale, then stay off it.

Reality: You can get rid of *anxiety* about the scale. Understanding the myths about scale usage, and actually weighing yourself every day will do that. And there are more tools and ideas later on in this book that can help with scale anxiety.

But there's going to be *some* emotion around your weight. There has to be, for your daily morning weigh-in to help you make better decisions every day.

It doesn't need to be traumatic. But you'll think something like "Good, I did okay yesterday", or "Darn, I need a better strategy for restaurant meals". Or even, "Well, I've been eating fine, but my weight is up because I haven't had a bowel movement. I won't worry about it."

For instance, imagine that you're up a pound that morning, and you know it's because you ate at a Chinese restaurant last night, without using good restaurant strategies. There's no need to be anxious, but now you know you need to work on that.

Maybe you'll make a strategy for eating fewer calories when you're eating out. Or perhaps you decide to limit restaurants to once a week. You may decide to balance heavy restaurant meals by eating less the next day.

You're the one who has to make those kinds of decisions. And more importantly—you will, because of the nudge of the daily weigh-in.

Myth: From a health perspective, the scale is not the best barometer. It gives you one piece of information, rather than the whole picture. If you want a clear understanding of what shape you're in, the simplest way is to get a physical.

Reality: Yes, the scale gives you one piece of information, but for most of us, it's the most useful one. What's the most common health problem in the United States, causing by far the most illness? Obesity.

There are other bits of health information that are useful, such as cholesterol levels and blood pressure. But these measures change very slowly when you're losing weight. Your actual weight can change more quickly. Imagine that you lose five pounds. That's an accomplishment, and it's very easy to see on the scale. But it would probably not change your cholesterol levels and blood pressure.

And, a physical, at a doctor's office, is very expensive, and done at most once a year. There's no way this could help motivate you, every day.

Myth: Weighing yourself every day is too much. You're turning your weight into a hobby, and you have better things to do with your life.

Reality: If we were living 100 years ago, then sure. Weighing yourself every day would be a waste of time, because most people were not overweight or obese. And the risk of becoming overweight or obese was low. We weren't constantly surrounded by cheap, delicious, high-calorie foods.

But we're not living 100 years ago. We're living in today's world, where the percentage of adult that are overweight or obese is over 71%. So almost 3 out of 4 people are overweight or obese. In the food environment we live in, it makes sense to watch our weight.

Most people brush their teeth at least once every day, to keep them healthy. Nobody would accuse you of having tooth-brushing as a hobby just because you brush your teeth regularly.

Stepping on the scale is a lot faster than brushing your teeth, and helps you lose weight, or keep your weight steady. Living in the current food environment, it makes sense.

Myth: "I've witnessed how upset people can get after stepping on a scale. There are people who regularly cry over their weight. As a culture, we have gotten it all wrong: Allowing a piece of metal to dictate how you feel about yourself is harming you in the long term."

Reality: The person writing this is a weight-loss counselor. If she doesn't get clients who like what she's saying, she'll be out of business.

There are countless weight loss counselors trying to drum up business for themselves, who will tell potential customers what they want to hear. And here's what many potential customers, struggling and anxious about their weight, want to hear:

- Weight doesn't matter.
- Weighing yourself regularly is a bad idea.
- The number on the scale is meaningless.

Try it yourself. Search online for the phrases "ditch your scale", "trash your scale", or "dump your scale". You'll find many, many articles written by people who are selling their counseling services.

They may be empathetic, kind people who truly believe what they're saying. But they make a living by selling counseling services on an hourly basis. They're going to promote what makes sense for their business.

These people have done their homework. There's definitely a group of potential customers who really want to be told that weight doesn't matter, and that you should throw away your scale. Articles like these have comments such as "Bless you a thousand times for writing this" and "Thanks for this post, it's exactly what I needed to hear!"

It's obvious that many people want to hear that weight doesn't matter. But that doesn't make it true, and it doesn't make throwing away the scale a good idea.

What I'm here to tell you is—of course the number on the scale doesn't determine your value. And I'm not here to say that you *should* lose weight. That's entirely your decision.

But what I am here to say is that *if* you've decided to lose weight, you should weigh yourself daily. Avoiding a daily weigh-in will make weight loss much harder.

Myth: It's useless to weigh yourself at home. Don't do it. Sign up for our expensive weight-loss program, and we will weigh you at our weekly sessions.

Reality: A friend of mine, Abby, signed up for a very expensive weight loss counseling program. There were some pre-packaged meals, plus a weekly session which included a weigh-in, listening to motivational tapes and personal counseling. And Abby was told again and again to *never* weigh herself at home. She was told that weigh-ins should happen *only* at their office.

Why is this? Why do all these companies want you to only weigh yourself once a week, in their office, on their scales?

I'm cynical about this. I believe that if you weigh yourself once a week as part of a program, instead of daily at home, it gets more emotional. If you've lost weight, your counselor will give you a smile and congratulate you. If you've gained weight, your counselor will offer some sympathy and encouragement for the next week.

Either way, by focusing on weighing in *only* at their office, on their scale, once a week, they're doing two things:

- **Creating a "Moment of Truth"**, for which they provide emotional support. It makes you feel grateful to them, either for their support and sympathy, or for their congratulations. They're trying to create an emotional bond.
- **Giving *them* ownership of *your* weight**. It's at their office, it's their scale, they record it in their system. I've heard many people say that they don't trust the scales at home, they only trust the ones at Weight Watchers.

Both of these are pushing you in the wrong direction.

The weigh-in should *not* be a "Moment of Truth". It's a daily tool to nudge you towards better decisions. Why do you need this nudge? Because we all live in a food environment that is *constantly* tempting us with delicious foods that—over the long run—lead to unhealthy bodies.

And the person who needs to own your weight is *you*. What happens when you allow someone else to weigh you, on their scale, on their schedule, in their system? It takes away ownership and responsibility from you.

It might feel more comfortable to "share" the responsibility for your weight. But it's your body. You make the choices, and you face the consequences. The more you take ownership and responsibility, the better your long-term outcome will be.

Myth: The most common reason people give for weighing every day is to "keep an eye on weight gain". But why haven't you adopted a *lifestyle* that will prevent this from happening? You need a *lifestyle eating plan* so you don't constantly have to worry about your weight

Reality: Weighing yourself every day is a smart thing to do, in the food environment we live in. The rate of obesity is going up all the time. The truth is that *most* people are gaining weight.

And guess what the person who wrote this is selling? A lifestyle eating plan. This is another example of people cynically pushing bad advice—bad advice that people *really* want to hear—to market their products.

Myth: Any time you feel weak or vulnerable, postpone weighing yourself for at least a day or two. Stay off the scale until you get back into a healthy balance, both physically and emotionally.

Reality: This only makes sense is if you see stepping on the scale as a *punishment*. Why would you want to punish yourself when you're feeling vulnerable?

But weighing yourself every day is *not* a punishment. It's a tool, a daily habit that makes weight loss and maintenance easier.

Avoiding the scale just because you're not feeling your best is a fast slide down a slippery slope. Say you "feel vulnerable" and don't step on the scale that day. Once you've done that, you're much less likely to step on the scale tomorrow, and the next day. You're more likely to overeat, because you've given yourself a way out. You can always just say, "I feel vulnerable—I'm going to postpone stepping on the scale."

The answer, in this situation, is *not* to delay weighing yourself. The answer is to understand:

- Why daily weigh-ins are one of the best health habits you can have

- The normal ups and downs that can happen with your weight, and why they happen
- How staying away from the scale causes *more* anxiety in the long run

And of course—keep weighing yourself every day!

Myth: Be sure to allow your body a few days to get back to its normal balance after a holiday party, or your mother's birthday dinner. The same thing applies after holiday meals such as Thanksgiving. The "day after" is not the time to see how much you weigh.

Reality: It's normal for your weight to be up after an event like a birthday dinner. Celebrations like this, that involve eating more than normal, can be a wonderful part of life.

But deliberately *avoiding* the scale the day after is a bad idea. You need to understand how your weight goes up and down as a result of what you ate and drank in the past few days.

And it can be a slippery slope. How much is "a few days"? When would you feel comfortable stepping on the scale again? In a day, a week, a month? Maybe never?

Instead of avoiding discomfort, realize that you have a valuable lifetime habit—stepping on the scale daily. Don't endanger this habit.

Just do it. This habit is a tool *you* have chosen. Remember, knowledge is power, and ignorance is *not* bliss.

Myth: Never weigh yourself right after a vacation. Right after a vacation, you'll nearly always see a false jump in your weight.

Reality: Instead of a "false" jump in weight, vacations often lead to permanent weight gains. Just like during the holiday season, during vacations people often eat more than normal. It may be just a few pounds, but sometimes they don't lose this weight. And this can lead to slow weight gain, every year. Awareness about weight gain is the first step to figuring out how to combat it.

It's very true that during travel and vacation, there are more random weight fluctuations. Traveling in a plane can cause water retention. And being outside your normal routine can cause your bathroom habits to be off. Both of these will cause your weight to be higher.

But there's also real weight gain that happens during travel and vacation. You're probably eating many meals in restaurants, and not cooking for yourself. These factors can cause you to eat many more calories than normal.

Weight fluctuations during travel and vacation are not reasons to avoid the scale. Consider packing a travel bathroom scale, and weigh yourself daily during your vacation. They're small, convenient, and accurate. If you don't do that, then you should definitely weigh yourself as soon as you get home. Your daily weigh-in habit is very valuable—don't put it at risk by making exceptions for travel and vacations.

Myth: Your weight fluctuates too much to make weighing yourself every day helpful.

Reality: Your weight can sometimes be higher than you're expecting, because of factors like water retention. There's a whole section earlier in this book, "Why your scale seems wrong sometimes" that goes through all the reasons this can happen.

But once you start weighing yourself daily, and observing the ups and downs that occur, you'll realize two things:

- A few of the fluctuations seem random, and hard to trace back to overeating.
- But most of the ups and downs are not random. They're related to what you ate and drank yesterday.

This second point is what will give you a nudge to make different choices. And those different choices, over the long term, are what can help you lose weight, or keep your weight steady.

Myth: Stepping on the scale every day is a bad idea, because muscle weighs more than fat. For instance, Arnold Schwarzenegger, in his bodybuilding prime, was technically overweight when he had almost no body fat.

Reality: There's a kernel of truth in this myth. It's true that some people with very low body fat could be classified as overweight, using standard charts. This is because of their muscle mass. These are people that are *very* highly muscled.

Here's how it gets distorted, though. Who are the people who are being misclassified as overweight? They're a tiny, elite group of athletes. They probably spend at least 2 hours a day, every day, in the gym, training and lifting weights.

If you're in this tiny, elite group of athletes, then you know who you are. You know that you're not overweight, and that instead you're extremely fit.

For everyone else—this is another myth to ignore.

The people pushing these myths above—they're telling you what you want to hear. They're telling you that weighing yourself daily is too stressful, so never weigh yourself. Or, weigh yourself only when you feel comfortable.

But for losing weight, this is not what you need. The first thing you need to do is to weigh yourself, *every single day*. It might not be comfortable at the beginning. But you should do it anyway. Developing the daily weigh-in habit will pay off in the long term.

Calorie counting—the pros and cons

What is calorie counting? Calorie counting is measuring and logging exactly what you're eating and drinking, and exactly how much. Calorie counting is often part of weight-loss programs. The theory is that if you control what you're eating and drinking by counting calories, you can't help but lose weight.

It's possible for calorie counting can be a very valuable part of your weight loss. But it's good to know the pros and cons before you make a commitment to it.

When you're counting calories, your log would look something like this:

Thursday, October 16

Breakfast

1 cup Cheerios	105 calories
½ cup whole milk	74 calories
½ banana	50 calories

Lunch

½ Red Robin Bacon Cheeseburger	525 calories
Red Robin house salad	110 calories
Unsweetened iced tea	5 calories
...and so on	

You'd keep a record like this for every meal, every day. And you would try to keep your daily calorie count under or at your target calorie count. Most people today count calories with an app on their phone. You write down what you're eating, and how much of it you're eating, and the app records the total calories.

Here's a best-case scenario. You're planning on eating one hard-boiled egg. You search for that in the food database that's part of the app, find it, log it and you're done.

But usually, it's much more complicated. Most of the time, unless you're specifically only eating foods that can be logged easily in your calorie counting app, it takes time. It could easily take much longer to track your food in the app than it would to prepare the food.

For instance, let's count the calories in your breakfast. Say you have a bowl of oatmeal for breakfast. You plan on cooking it with milk in the microwave, adding some raisins and chopped walnuts, and some peanut butter. That's a straightforward, healthy breakfast.

Now, try to log it in your calorie tracking app. I've used calorie counting apps before, but I tried one again just now, to refresh my memory on how much work it can be.

Here's the steps you need to do, before you can even start:

- **Choose which app to use**. Many of these apps exist, all with their own pros and cons. One app that I used years ago was fine back then. But since then it was bought by a different company which has flooded it with advertisements, making it a hassle to use.
- **Choose a pricing plan**. Most apps have a premium plan, and also a free version with annoying ads. Which should you choose?
- **Sign in and set up your account**. It turns out that one app I tried (My Fitness Pal) is one I've tried earlier. So, I couldn't use the same email, because I'd forgotten the password I used the last time. I couldn't reset my password, so I ended up needing to use a different email address.

Suppose we've completed all these steps, and everything is set up correctly. Now we're eager to start tracking what we've been eating and drinking. Here's an example of what you need to do, *every single time you eat or drink something*. This is based on me trying to log the healthy bowl of oatmeal I described above.

First, I'll start with the oatmeal. I started out by just pouring some oatmeal into my bowl, but of course that's a mistake—I need to pour out a measured amount. So, I have to empty the oatmeal back into the original container, take out a half-cup measure, and measure out exactly one half-cup of oatmeal into the bowl. From the looks of it, one-half cup is a little skimpy, but I don't want the hassle of having to measure out more, so I'll just leave it. Now—I'll enter that in the calorie counting app. So, I go to "Breakfast", and "Add Food", then "Search for a Food", then type "oatmeal".

There seems to be an endless number of choices for oatmeal. It's hard to figure out which one is just regular oatmeal. It looks like every grocery store and restaurant has a listing (Aldi, Trader Joe's, Panera, McDonald's), as well as every brand (Quaker, Walmart). Finally, I pick ½ cup of Aldi Oatmeal.

So, that's done. I now have a total of 150 calories. Only 4 more food (milk, raisins, chopped walnuts, peanut butter) to add!

I won't bore you with further descriptions of what a pain it is to measure and log all the foods in my simple, healthy breakfast. But I hope that this description is enough to show one thing—calorie counting may be simple (just log every calorie that passes your lips), but it is *not* easy. It's complicated, time-consuming, and requires lots of decision making.

Is it possible to make counting your calories easier? Sure. Here's some ways to make logging what you eat and drink more straightforward:

- **Eat the same foods, mostly**. Calorie counting apps usually have a feature where you can save a bunch of separate foods (like the oatmeal breakfast I mentioned above, with oatmeal, milk, raisins, chopped walnuts, and butter) together, as a "recipe". This makes it easier to log your regular meals, once you've done the work of setting them up. If your meals are very routine, this can be easy.
- **Eat more packaged, processed food**. Packaged foods have the total calories right on the label. Also, they're easy to find when you search in the calorie counting app. For instance, suppose I need to log that I ate a Peanut Butter Granola Clif Bar. I type in the whole name, and bingo, it comes right up.

The first option, eating mostly the same foods, can work well and be a healthy choice. If you have a specific, measured amount of foods that you're going to eat regularly, you can save it in the app, and it's easy to log the next time you eat the same thing.

The second option, of eating mostly packaged foods, is not a healthy choice, even though it makes make logging calories easier. I'll have more to say later about why avoiding packaged foods is important, but for now let's just note that the more packaged foods you eat, the less healthy your diet probably is.

So, we've settled that counting calories is a tremendous hassle. But *does it work*?

The bottom line is—yes. Many, many studies prove that dieters who accurately log what they're eating and drinking lose much more weight than those who don't. Dieters that log their daily calories 7 days a week lose more weight than those that do it 4 days a week. Dieters that measure and log their calories before they eat lose more weight than those that try to remember and log what they ate yesterday, or the day before.

So, there's a strong link between calorie counting and weight loss. But what happens in the real world, after the initial excitement of the weight loss? People can't keep up the habit, and they stop counting calories. They stop, because it's such a time-consuming, inconvenient thing to do. Almost nobody can make this a lifetime habit.

Some people use calorie counting and daily weigh-ins, together, as strategies for losing weight. And if you have the willpower to keep up the calorie counting, it can work great. The problem happens when you give calorie counting the same importance as logging your weight daily. But they're not equal.

Logging your weight daily—this should be the long-term, gold-plated, lifetime habit. But calorie counting is not. It's a short-term tool. It's can be very helpful, but it's a strategy, one of many strategies that you can use. And almost nobody will find it possible to count calories for a lifetime. It's just too much work.

Some people *are* able to use one set of habits (such as calorie counting), to get to a weight loss goal, and then successfully keep the weight off, even after they stop counting calories.

But some people aren't able to. Here's what can happen:

- You decide to lose weight.
- You adopt some short-term habits, such as calorie counting.
- These short-term habits lead to weight loss.
- Once you're at your goal weight, you congratulate yourself. You stop counting calories.
- Maintaining your weight is hard, because you've dropped the main habit (calorie counting) that was critical to your weight loss.
- You gradually gain your weight back.

This is a classic pattern. It can lead people to say that calorie counting just doesn't work.

The truth is that calorie counting *does* work, but it's hard to keep up. And switching from one strategy for losing weight, to another strategy for maintaining weight—that's difficult.

But let's say you completely understand that calorie counting is *not* going to be a lifetime habit. And you know it's *not* going to be your only tool for weight management. In this case, calorie counting can be very helpful.

I counted calories myself, for a while. I was having a hard time losing the weight I gained during pregnancy. So, I weighed myself daily, and I also logged the calories whenever I ate or drank anything. I used an app on my phone, and a food scale. I measured, weighed, and wrote down every single calorie, trying very hard to be accurate.

This is how I know, from personal experience, two things. Calorie counting works, if you have the time and motivation to be accurate. I lost the weight I wanted to.

The other thing I learned is that there's no way I could do it for a lifetime. It's a huge amount of work, and hard to fit into daily life. And after I stopped counting my calories, I started slowly gaining weight again.

Calorie counting gives you a good sense for how many calories are in your food. And that's very useful. Calories are *the* basic unit in nutrition. There's a lot of talk about good calories and bad calories; and the pros and cons of low-carb/high-fat diets. But the fact remains—the daily balance between *calories in* (what you eat and drink) to *calories out* (the amount of energy you use) is critical. This is what causes you to either lose weight, maintain weight, or gain weight.

I would never recommend that you track all your calories, for a lifetime. There may be some iron-willed people who can pull it off. But most people can't, or don't want to. It feels unnatural, and it's just far too much work.

However, weighing and measuring your food, and counting your calories for a limited period–a few weeks or months—can be very useful. It will give you an education in calorie awareness and portion size. The knowledge you gain from calorie counting—while understanding that it's not a lifetime habit—can be very valuable.

Summary

- Weighing yourself daily gives feedback about the habits that help you lose weight, and those that make you gain weight.
- Sometimes your weight can be up for reasons that aren't related to what you ate—for instance, water retention. But usually it's a reliable indicator of how you ate yesterday.
- Weighing yourself daily instead of weekly is much easier to keep up as a lifetime habit. You're less likely to forget, there's less anxiety, and you get the daily feedback you need.
- Weighing yourself should not be a "moment of truth" event. "Moment of truth" thinking causes stress and anxiety. It should be a daily habit, like brushing your teeth.
- There are many myths about weighing yourself daily. It's important to understand these myths, and the reality behind them.
- Calorie counting can be a very useful, temporary strategy for weight loss. As a long-term strategy, most people can't keep it up.

WEIGHING YOURSELF EVERY DAY: THE FUNDAMENTALS

---

*How to make this lifetime habit
simple and straightforward, and
ditch your anxiety about the scale*

We've all heard a lot of biased, inaccurate information about weighing yourself, and how often you should do it. I hope you're now convinced that stepping on the scale daily is one of the best health habits you can develop.

Even so, those old beliefs can still cause doubts and confusion. This chapter will go through the fundamentals of weighing yourself every day, and how to make it straightforward and painless. There should be no barriers to weighing yourself every day, either mental or physical.

What kind of scale should I buy?

You can buy a cheap, accurate digital bathroom scale now for under $30. If you don't have one, go out and buy one now, or order it online.

I recommend a simple scale that measures one thing—your weight. It should have a large, easy-to-read display. There's lots of scales that claim to measure other things, such as body fat. And some will attempt to tell you your water weight, muscle weight, etc.

All of these additional numbers are distracting and unnecessary. Body fat measurements based on a step-on scale are known for being inaccurate. They can also fool you into being dishonest with yourself. You might think, "My weight is going up or staying the same, but my body fat measurement looks good, so I must be doing well."

No. Just stick with the one number—your weight. That's enough, and it's simple to track. Remember, the scale is your honest, blunt friend.

I recommend a digital bathroom scale with *no* additional features. That means no Bluetooth enabled scales, no memory/weight tracking on the scale. You just need one simple number—your weight.

The reason I advocate no additional features is that they can cause problems and distractions. Also, a scale that does many things—Bluetooth, body fat measurements, memory or weight tracking—will not be as accurate as a basic scale. You need a scale that just measures one thing.

What you need is simplicity. Suppose you have a Bluetooth enabled scale, that sends you a daily email when you weigh yourself. Everything may work fine for a while, but then you have a problem

84

with the Bluetooth feature on the scale. It gives you an error message. Are you going to try to find the customer service number for the scale manufacturer, and try to contact them? Are you going to search online to find the answer yourself?

Fixing this kind of problem is a hassle. And if you don't fix it right away, it may be an excuse to give up the habit of weighing yourself daily.

After a year or so, you will have a rock-solid daily habit of weighing yourself. You plan and *know* you will keep up this habit for a lifetime. Once you've reached this point, feel free to experiment with different scales and features. But for now, keep it very simple.

Where should I put the scale?

The scale belongs in the bathroom, on a solid surface floor, and not on a rug or carpet. It should be visible and easy to access. Make room for it right on your way to the shower or tub, without making it a trip hazard.

Never put it underneath something like a cabinet or shelf, where you need to pull it out to use it. Unless your scale is easy to get to, and something you walk past every morning, you simply won't use it. When you're establishing a daily habit, convenience should be a top priority.

When should I weigh myself?

You should weigh yourself daily, after you wake up, after emptying your bladder, with no clothes on. Maybe right before you step into the shower is the best time for you. In the morning, you'll be at your most stable and lowest weight of the day.

If you're honestly forgetting to weigh yourself—not avoiding the scale because of anxiety, but simply forgetting—then try taping a reminder note on your shower door. Or maybe it would be better to put your toothpaste on the scale as a reminder, assuming you brush your teeth every morning. The bottom line is, do whatever works best for *your* individual morning routine. You need to make stepping on the scale daily a well-established habit, one that's easy to do and impossible to forget.

If you happen to forget to weigh yourself in the morning, don't wait to weigh yourself the next morning. Just step on the scale as soon as you can. Don't worry about removing all your clothes. Your weight will be higher than it normally would be. But it'll be a reminder to do it in the morning tomorrow. And it's extremely important to establish the daily habit and routine of weighing yourself, without excuses.

Remember, the scale is your honest, blunt friend. But it can only help you if you use it regularly.

Logging your weight—an important part of your daily weigh-in

When you weigh yourself every day, what do you do with that number? Do you just keep it in your head? Or should you write it down?

My advice is—write it down. Writing down your weight daily, just after you weigh yourself, helps you lose weight, and helps you maintain your weight. Here's how it can help.

Writing it down helps you remember

Once you've written down your weight, it's easier to remember. Physically tracking a measurement makes you notice it. And knowing your weight helps counteract the constant stimulation of food around us—the sight and smell of delicious, unhealthy foods. It helps you say "No" to that big leftover tray of donuts in the office. It reminds you to plan ahead for lunch, instead of doing whatever is easiest at the moment.

You can track your progress

Having a steady, daily record of your weight allows you to track your progress, and see patterns. For instance, you may see that you don't lose weight, or even gain weight, on weekends. Information like this can help you decide how to adjust your eating habits. The decisions are all yours, but writing down and tracking your weight helps you find patterns.

Seeing progress over time is deeply satisfying

Once you've been logging your weight for a while, you'll have a chart of your progress. Hopefully, you'll be seeing one of two patterns:

- Slow, steady weight loss, based on habit changes that you've made.
- Steady weight maintenance, with minor ups and downs. You've lost the weight you want to lose, and will be maintaining that for a lifetime.

Either way, you've had the courage and self-awareness to weigh yourself daily, and log that number. That's a big accomplishment, and it can be very rewarding to see this on your weight chart.

Weight gain is more obvious

Suppose you've completed your weight loss, and you're maintaining your weight. You're logging your weight daily on graph paper that has a 10-pound range, from 175 to 185. This is what you've decided is your healthy range for you.

Guess what? If you're 186 or over, there's no place to log your weight! You'll have to scribble a note on the top margin.

This is a good thing, though. This forces you to face reality sooner. You know you need to make changes. And small weight gains are so much easier to fix. The large weight gains that you will get if you ignore the problem—those are much more difficult.

How to log your weight

Logging your weight daily is a habit you need to keep up for a lifetime, just like stepping on the scale is a lifetime habit.

What does this mean? It means that you need to make this habit easy, and straightforward.

You brush your teeth every day, so you wouldn't keep your toothbrush inconveniently tucked away in your closet. The same principle applies to your scale, and how you log your weight. The scale needs to be noticeable and very easy to access. And writing down your weight needs to take no thought, and almost no time.

In my bathroom, the scale is right next to the shower, so I step past it before showering. It's impossible to miss. I have a sheet of graph paper taped to the wall above the scale, just at eye level. My pencil is tied to a string, which is taped to the wall next to my weight chart. There's no searching for a special notebook, or looking for a pencil. The whole process of stepping on the scale and logging my weight takes me less than 4 seconds.

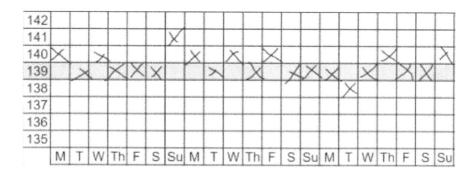

Here's what my weight chart looks like currently. Since I'm just working on maintaining my weight around 139, I have a narrow range on my chart. The row for 139 is highlighted, since that's the weight I want to be around. And instead of writing down a number, I just have the graph paper set up as you see above. So, I just mark an "X" in the square for that number.

Here's what a weight chart could look like, for someone who's actively working on losing weight, and starting at a weight of around 210 pounds.

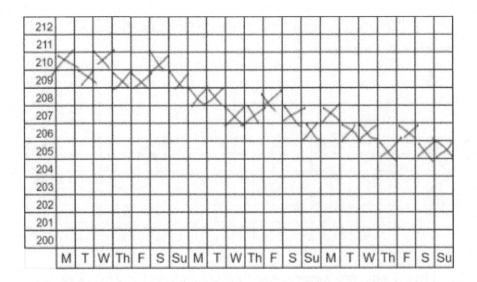

This shows a weight loss of between one and two pounds a week, which can be a reasonable pace. This pace of weight loss, or less, is what you can expect when you're slowly changing your food habits.

It's very satisfying to see a slow, steady decrease in your weight on the graph paper. Or, if you're working on maintaining your weight—seeing that "X" for your weight stay in the same range feels good. When you're marking the number on a graph, instead of just writing down a number, changes become very obvious. Just a glance will show if you're going up, down, or staying steady.

You can buy some graph paper at the store to make your weight chart, or print out some graph paper online (search for "printable graph paper"). Or you could make them yourself with a spreadsheet such as Excel or Google Sheets. But to start, all you really need is a sheet of graph paper and a pencil. You can also download weight charts at my website, WeighEveryDay.com.

You may want to make a line on your paper at your short-term goal weight. Say you have a short-term goal of losing 5 pounds.

90

Make a line at that number, going across the graph. Or you could mark a line pointing downward, that shows your target weight loss. A reasonable weight loss might be about one pound a week, or two pounds a month.

The actual process of stepping on the scale and logging your weight needs to be as easy and straightforward as possible. That's because any bumps in the road can make it hard to keep up the habit of weighing yourself, every day. And weighing yourself every day should be the foundation of your weight loss and weight maintenance. It's what keeps you on track. It needs to be completely foolproof and convenient.

What about tracking your weight in an app? I suggest that you avoid it. Some of the popular, heavily marketed weight loss apps are expensive and not very user-friendly. Plus, some of them don't let you see your weight history—the history that *you* entered—once you stop paying for the subscription.

You're better off just taping a piece of paper to the wall, and logging your weight on it. It's simple and foolproof. You won't need to pay anything, or login. You don't need your phone or a computer. You can save the graph paper with the record of your weight on it— nothing fancy needed, just put them in an envelope or notebook.

If you want to get more technical, I suggest that you to still log your weight on a piece of paper, but once a month, transfer it to a spreadsheet. That way you could do fancy things like a moving average of your weight, various graphs and charts, etc. But that part is completely optional.

Some people recommend using a Bluetooth scale that communicates with an app on your phone. They say you shouldn't even look at your weight, that you should look only at a 10-day moving average, which will smooth out daily changes.

I say—no. That just makes the whole setup too complex. Once you've overcome your anxiety about stepping on the scale, just keep it simple. The simpler it is, the more likely you'll keep it up for a lifetime. Complexity like Bluetooth scales, apps on your phone, moving averages, etc., are just more places for problems to happen. And these problems could give you an excuse to give up your daily weigh-in habit.

But the bottom line is—*you* know yourself best. If you know that you'd do better with a more complex scale that connects with your phone, then do that. If you'd rather log your weight on a spreadsheet, instead of a piece of graph paper taped to your wall, then do what works for you.

What's most important is that you weigh yourself every day, log it somehow, and keep that habit up for a lifetime.

Make your personal "Why I want to lose weight" list

Your initial weight loss goal could be 5 pounds, or 10. Or it may be to get below a certain target weight—say 200 pounds. These numeric goals are very motivating. But another strong motivator that you should take advantage of is knowing *your* personal reasons for losing weight. Make a list of these reasons, and keep them handy.

Some generic reasons to lose weight are:

- To have less joint pain
- To avoid a higher risk of heart disease
- To sleep better

These may be great reasons to lose weight—but are they motiving for you? Be honest with yourself. Come up with the reasons that you, specifically, want to lose weight. These might be reasons like:

- My knees hurt when I walk. I know that if I lost some weight, I'd feel better
- I want to get pregnant. My doctor told me that if I lost 20 pounds, I'd have a much better chance.
- I want to lose weight to make it easier to travel by plane. Right now, I worry about needing a seatbelt extender, and crowding the people next to me.
- I worry that I'm not setting a good example for my kids. Plus, if I lost weight, I'd be able to get up and down from the floor more easily, to play with them.
- Summer is coming up, and I want to wear a swimsuit that looks good.
- My doctor told me that I'm pre-diabetic, and need to lose weight unless I want to give myself insulin shots for the rest of my life.
- I want to find a boyfriend/girlfriend.

Reasons like these are immediate, very personal, and more motivating to you than reasons like "to avoid a higher risk of heart disease". Sure, heart disease and stroke are some of the most serious risks of being overweight, but they're also in the far-off future.

93

Write your "Why I want to lose weight" list on an index card, and update it when you think of more reasons. Put it in your pocket and read it daily. Or perhaps put it on the wall next to your weight chart, where you see it every day as you log your weight. Do whatever works best for you.

Anxiety over weighing yourself, and how to overcome it

You may be completely, 100% on-board with weighing yourself daily, as a lifetime habit. If so—well done! Developing the mindset that you *will* keep up this daily routine, forever, deserves a pat on the back.

But you may still have some anxiety about stepping on the scale. Many people do. Maybe you haven't done it in a long time. Perhaps you know it will show you a number that you don't want to see.

Here's the thing, though. The number—your weight—exists even if you don't know it. It exists, and it affects your health. Not paying attention to it, or telling yourself it doesn't matter, is a bad idea over the long run.

For people with weight problems, the most common outcome of not weighing yourself for weeks or months at a time is weight gain. Here's some comments taken from an article on weight, in the UK newspaper The Guardian:

***

Every time I have gained massive amounts of weight, I was not weighing myself.

94

I now weigh myself every morning before breakfast. Over the last 8 months I have lost 41lbs. It is crucial feedback that I rely on.

✳✳✳

I have battery operated digital scales in my bathroom. I didn't replace the battery when it gave out, and when I finally replaced it about six months later, I was shocked to discover that I'd gained about 7lbs without really noticing.

✳✳✳

Deliberately ignoring your weight, while knowing that it's going up and up, is stressful. Ignoring reality doesn't help. What helps is getting up the courage to face it.

Also, you should know that you do *not* need to make changes to your eating habits immediately. Just getting comfortable with stepping on the scale daily, and deciding that you'll do that for a lifetime—that's a huge accomplishment. Don't underestimate it. Many people spend a few weeks or more, just weighing themselves daily, and getting comfortable with that routine, without doing anything else.

If you're anxious about stepping on the scale, below are some ways to work through that anxiety. Read through the following tips, and see if one or more of them will help you overcome your concerns.

Prepare yourself mentally

You may want to review the chapter "Why weighing yourself daily is essential". Take some notes. If you have a solid

95

understanding of the evidence supporting a daily weigh-in habit, it'll be much easier to follow.

Get comfortable with the scale

Play with it. Turn it on, and weigh some larger items on the scale. It'll have to be something heavier, like for instance a potted plant, since most bathroom scales have a minimum of 20 pounds.

You may never be 100% comfortable with the scale. But doing things that are uncomfortable is a part of life. If you avoid everything that's hard, you'll miss out on much of life.

Consider weighing yourself in kilograms instead of pounds

Or pounds instead of kilograms—whichever one is less familiar to you. Most modern digital scales have an option (usually a switch at the bottom) to switch between kilograms and pounds.

Obviously, your weight will still be the same, whether it's expressed in kilograms or pounds. But—if you're worried about whether you're above or below a certain trigger number—maybe 200 pounds—then switching to kilograms may not be as stressful. And it will be just as accurate. You can switch back to pounds (or kilograms) later on.

Before getting on the scale, drink some water

Give yourself some time to drink a couple glasses of water, before you step on the scale for the first time in a long while.

Or, weigh yourself, write down how much you weigh, then drink a few glasses of water and weigh yourself again.

Notice that your weight has gone up because of the water. It'll probably have increased at least a pound or two. Obviously, the water has no calories, so it's a change that has no long-term effects.

This helps reinforce the idea that stepping on the scale is not a "moment of truth". It's a number. But knowing that number can be essential for getting to a healthy weight range, and staying in that range.

Put a piece of masking tape on the display of the scale

You may want to give yourself a few days of just stepping on the scale, and getting used to it, without actually knowing your weight. So, put a piece of masking tape on the display. Doing this for a few days can help you adjust to the habit, if you've had anxiety about it.

Hold something heavy in your hands while stepping on the scale

If you're still feeling reluctant to step on the scale, fill up a few water bottles or milk jugs, hold them in your hands, and then weigh yourself. Or use a handheld weight, like a dumbbell. If you do this, you will know that the weight you see is not just your weight, it's also whatever you're holding in your hands.

∗∗∗

It's all about getting more comfortable stepping on the scale. You may need to work up to it gradually, and that's fine. As long as you get to the point where you have a firm commitment to a lifetime daily weigh-in habit, you're doing great.

Some of the tips I've given above could be considered "systematic desensitization". This is the name of a psychological treatment designed to help people get rid of fears and phobias. It's also one of the most well-proven psychological treatments.

Here's how it works. Suppose you have anxiety about dogs. You could slowly work your way towards getting comfortable with dogs by going through these steps, with or without a therapist.

- Looking at pictures of dogs
- Watching a video of dogs
- Standing across the street from a leashed dog
- Petting a puppy held by someone else
- Petting a larger dog

Gradually, step by step, your anxiety about dogs will be overcome.

You can take gradual steps, similar to this, if you have anxiety about getting on the scale. It's something that you *can* overcome, with or without a therapist.

It can be hard, because sometimes the scale delivers news that you don't want to hear. And nobody likes a messenger who delivers bad news. So, you may have anxiety when you first start stepping on the scale. But you can overcome it. Remember, the scale is your honest, blunt friend.

When you're trying to lose weight, knowing that number every day is essential to figuring out if your strategies are working. And when you're maintaining your weight, you need to know immediately if the number goes up. Then you can adjust quickly.

Waiting until you "feel like it" is a losing strategy when deciding how often to step on the scale. Get used to weighing yourself every single day. You *will* get used to it, and it *will* get easier.

Overcoming other obstacles

Travel and vacations

There are times where it's inconvenient to weigh yourself daily. Anytime that you're out of your normal daily routine can be hard—for instance, vacations, and visiting friends and family. Even people that have lost a lot of weight, reached their goal weight, and have kept it up for *years* have difficulty when they're not able to weigh themselves daily.

> During the honeymoon, and later while staying with his wife's family, Chris didn't have access to a scale. This proved disastrous. He knew he was gaining weight—he could feel it—but without the scale, it was impossible to gauge exactly how much he was gaining. Without the daily reminder that he was overeating, it was impossible for him to refuse temptation.
> —The Economist's Diet

Chris Payne, one of the co-authors of The Economist's Diet, stepped on the scale after his honeymoon and realized that he had gained 10 pounds. And this was after he had lost a large chunk of weight, and kept off that weight for 18 months. It was frustrating, but he started stepping on the scale every day again, got back on track, and lost those 10 pounds within 2 months.

This story illustrates a few points:

- Maintaining your weight during travel can be really difficult
- Stepping on the scale daily is very important. Even if you *know* you're gaining weight, it's easier to ignore if you don't know the number.
- This applies to everyone, even to people who have successfully kept their weight off for a long time. Knowing your weight—the actual number—can give you a reason to say "no" to temptation.

During travel, you're even more vulnerable to weight gain. Not only because you're away from your scale but because your routine is out of whack, and you're probably eating much more restaurant food. If you're on a cruise, or an all-inclusive resort, you may be constantly tempted with all-you-can-eat buffets of the most appetizing foods that exist.

Here's the good news. There are inexpensive, travel-sized bathroom scales that are just as accurate as regular-sized scales. I have one, and often take it on trips. It's tiny and lightweight, about the dimensions of a sheet of paper folded in half, but thicker.

Bringing a travel scale on trips may seem like overkill. I would have called it extreme myself, a few years ago. But that was before I realized how out of whack our food environment is, and how easy it is to gain weight when you're not weighing yourself daily.

Ten or twenty years ago, the weight I gained during travel or visits to family came off again without much effort. I regularly gained a few pounds during trips. That extra weight would disappear in a few weeks, almost without effort.

But as the decades pile on, as you exit your 20's and get into your 30's, 40's and beyond—things change. Your body changes. The small weight gains, the ones that easily vanished a decade ago—they stay with you. Most people aren't paying attention, and end up gradually gaining weight over the years.

To avoid this, the first thing to do is to know your weight. Track your weight. I highly recommend bringing a travel-sized digital bathroom scale on trips. This may be even more important if you're on a type of trip where most people gain weight, like a cruise.

Your weight may fluctuate more than normal when traveling. That's because we eat differently when we travel—we eat out more, we eat fewer fruits and vegetables, and more greasy fried foods. So, expect your weight to fluctuate more. But you don't need to stop your habit of weighing yourself.

Shared bathrooms

Another common obstacle to logging your weight daily is sharing your bathroom. You may not want whoever you're sharing a bathroom with—spouse, boyfriend or girlfriend, or roommate—to see your weight.

You can deal with this situation in a few different ways. Some are obvious, like writing your weight in a little private notebook, instead of in a chart on the wall.

But here's a suggestion. Think about this situation:

Melissa and Michelle are roommates, and share a bathroom. Melissa is trying to lose weight, and wants to weigh herself every day, and log her weight on a chart above the scale. She's not happy to do this in a place that she shares with someone else—the shared bathroom. She'd rather keep her weight private.

Here's two potential scenarios:

- Melissa is uncomfortable logging her weight daily in the shared bathroom, but she does it anyway.
- Melissa is uncomfortable logging her weight daily in the shared bathroom, so she moves the scale to her own room, and tries to weigh herself daily and log her weight there.

In which of these two scenarios will Melissa be more successful in managing her weight?

The answer is clear. In the first scenario, Melissa has faced a little discomfort (having her weight visible to her roommate). She may have felt awkward the first week or so, but she overcome it, because she realized the most convenient place for the scale was the bathroom. And convenience is critical when establishing a lifetime habit.

So, I suggest that you overcome the awkwardness, and log your weight in a shared bathroom anyway.

But as I've mentioned before—my suggestions are not the only way to do things. Weighing yourself daily is essential, and logging your weight is important, but *you* know yourself best. You may decide to keep the scale in the bathroom next to the shower, but log it in a more private place.

Should you tell people you plan to lose weight?

Many people believe that the more people that know about your goal, the more it will motivate and help them. The more accountability the better, right? So, you should do things like tell everyone your weight-loss plans and goals, and hire a weight-loss coach, to "keep you accountable".

Well, it may work for you. You are the best judge of that, and you may have a system that works for you. But based on my experiences and what I've seen and heard, accountability can be a double-edged sword. Adding accountability can be useless. It can make things more complicated. And keeping your goals private can be more helpful than shouting them from the rooftops.

Of course, having supportive family or friends can be valuable. Having someone that shares healthy recipes, and takes walks with you, is obviously helpful. But when you rely on other people for *accountability*, that's different. Relying on other people for accountability can actually make you *less* likely to achieve your goal.

Here's why.

Having someone to be "accountable" to often decreases your feeling of ownership and responsibility. For instance, say you go to the gym to meet a trainer for a workout. And since you've paid for the trainer, and have someone waiting for you at the gym, this gives you a push to actually go there, and not put it off.

What could go wrong with this?

Plenty. Here's what I've seen. A friend of mine had a hard time getting himself to the gym. Something always seemed to get in the way. Or he was tired. So, he hired a personal trainer who worked at the gym. He met with this same trainer for *two years*, three times a week. The trainer would tell him what to do, and lead him through exercises. He spent *a lot* of money on his personal trainer.

So, he exercised regularly for two years. That was good.

But here's what was bad. He never took personal responsibility. If my friend had been exercising on his own, he probably would have figured out how to make it more convenient and enjoyable. Maybe he would have set up a home workout routine, to avoid the half-hour drive to the gym. But he had hired the personal trainer to "keep him accountable". So, he didn't do anything himself except show up at the gym, and do what the trainer told him.

Then the personal trainer moved to another city. My friend had plenty of opportunities to switch to another trainer, and was encouraged to do so. But he didn't. Instead, he stopped working out. Having a personal trainer—for two years—did not help him develop the motivation to work out on his own. Working out was always a hassle, and he got through it by having someone else take responsibility. And when there was a little bump in the road—his trainer left—he dropped the habit entirely.

✳✳✳

Another consequence of making your goals public, is that you'll get plenty of kudos. People will congratulate you. They'll say things like, "Hey, that's awesome! You go, girl!"

This sounds great. You're being encouraged, and given supportive feedback. What could go wrong?

Potentially, lots. It often happens that the more you're congratulated on *starting* a goal, or *intending* to do something, the less likely that you'll actually do it. This is not the case for everyone—it may not be the case for you—but you should know that it happens often.

What tends to occur is that sharing your goal is not the first step to achieving your goal. Instead, it becomes a *substitute* for achieving your goal. You get so much positive feedback for announcing a goal, that your subconscious mind thinks, "Hey, I'm already halfway done. Not much need to work on it anymore."

Also, what are the chances that a friend of yours is ever going to say, "Hey, about that goal you posted on Facebook six months ago, to lose 20 pounds—what happened with that? Did you actually lose 20 pounds?" Unless you have unusual friends, that won't happen.

✳✳✳

Here's another story. A friend of mine—I'll call her Nicole—wanted to lose weight. She paired up with a friend living in another state. The plan was that they would send each other a daily photo of the read-out from a digital scale. They would encourage and support each other, as their weight dropped off.

It didn't work out. After a week of photo exchanges, the daily sending of the scale photo was occasionally skipped, with no consequences. And when Nicole's friend didn't send a daily photo, Nicole didn't feel as obligated to send a photo the following day. A few more days were missed because of business travel or vacation.

And that's how the plan died. Neither of them felt like being an enforcer of the rules. They were good friends, after all. It would have felt like they were being harsh. Neither of them wanted to say, "Hey! You didn't step on the scale and send me a photo yesterday!" But that meant that the rules didn't get enforced.

Is there a better way to do this type of thing? Probably. And you may discover an accountability system that truly works for you.

But the bottom line is, you should be skeptical of the idea that "accountability" is always better. Maybe it is, maybe it isn't. The reality is that you can rely on yourself. You are the one who will gain the benefits of losing weight, and you are the one who has to do the work.

Action Step Checklist

_____ I have a quality digital bathroom scale.

_____ My scale is convenient to use—I walk by it every morning.

_____ I've decided when, exactly, to weigh myself every morning (for instance, "just before I step into the shower").

_____ I've made a firm commitment to weigh myself every morning.

_____ I have a weight chart taped to the wall, or some other easy way of logging my weight.

_____ I've made my personal "Why I want to lose weight" list.

_____ If I feel anxious about weighing myself, I've taken some steps to overcome that.

_____ I have a plan for watching my weight during travel and vacations, which may include a travel scale.

DIET AND FOOD MYTHS

*Don't let these myths distract you
from the habit changes you need
to make*

Before antibiotics were developed, getting an infection could be a
death sentence. People regularly died of infections that would be
considered trivial today. And there were many different treatments
for infections, such as blood-letting, herbal medicines, and toxic
ingredients such as mercury.

These types of infections, before antibiotics, were a very difficult
and serious problem. No reliable treatment existed. And specifically
because nothing was very successful, many different treatments
existed. If you don't have a good solution to a serious problem,
people are willing to try anything. But none of them really worked
well.

And then antibiotics came along. All the other treatments for infections were abandoned as soon as antibiotics became available. Antibiotics were the first "miracle drug".

You're probably asking yourself—what does this have to do with dieting and weight loss?

Here's the thing. We now have a very similar situation with dieting and weight loss. Obesity is a massive problem, affecting more and more people every year. It's similar to what bacterial infections were years ago, in terms of how serious the problem is.

But there's no clear solution to the obesity problem. The miracle drug hasn't arrived yet. There's no equivalent of antibiotics. And because of this gap, many different myths are spread. People want to hear *some* kind of solution, even if it ends up being wrong—as long as it promises to fix the problem.

In this chapter, I'm going to go through some of the most popular food and diet myths. Looking carefully at these myths will help you clear your mind. The less time you spend worrying about things that don't matter (like whether you should eat low-carb), the more time you have to work on what really does matter.

Low-carb/Paleo diet

The most popular diet now is the low-carb diet. It's gone through many different versions, and currently, what's popular is the Paleo version of the low-carb diet. Some of the previous versions of the low-carb diet are the Atkins diet, the Stillman diet, and going back more than a century, the Banting diet.

So, low-carb diets have been around a long, long time. At the core of all low-carb diets is to drastically limit complex carbohydrates such as bread, pasta, potatoes; and to eliminate most sugar.

The Paleo version of the low-carb diet is that we should all eat the same foods as our very distant "paleolithic" ancestors ate. Fans of the Paleo diet assume this includes mostly meat and leafy vegetables, and no starchy foods like grains or potatoes, no legumes, and no dairy.

Paleo Diet	
Good foods	**Bad foods**
Coconut oil	Oatmeal
Avocado	Bread
Butter	Milk
Grass-fed meats	Potatoes
Some vegetables	Beans
Almonds	Sugar

I'm not going to get into lots of specific details of the Paleo diet. But it's a good example of a fad diet, one that has its day in the sun, and will then fade away, as so many other diets have in the past. Understanding why the Paleo diet isn't helpful over the long term helps us understand why most diets aren't helpful over the long term.

One good aspect of the Paleo diet was that in its original version, it was supposed to include no processed food. No chips, no desserts, etc. But what soon began to happen is that "Paleo-friendly" chips and desserts soon became available. If you search online for "Paleo Treats" you'll find all kinds of treats available. They have strange ingredients like tapioca flour, coconut flour, and other hard-to-find items.

Also, what the Paleo diet promises is that as long as you eat only what's allowed on the diet, you don't need to watch *how much* you eat. In other words, it's "all you can eat". But for most people, that ends up not being true at all. If you're eating mostly high-fat and high-protein foods, you *do* need to watch the quantities. Fat is calorie dense, and it's easy to overeat.

***

Does a low-carb, Paleo diet help you lose weight? It can. But that's not the issue. *All* diets help you lose weight, over the short term. A low-carb diet is just another form of diet that dramatically restricts a particular food group. And that type of diet will usually end up with you eating fewer calories. If you can't eat a major part of your normal diet—if bread, pasta, and dairy are all forbidden— then you will probably lose weight. That's not controversial.

Say you *are* able to lose weight on this diet. Then the issue becomes: can you stick to this diet? Can you eat a low-carb Paleo diet for the rest of your life? Or would it be just another very restrictive diet that you drop, because it's just too difficult to keep up?

That's what ends up happening with most people who are on a low-carb diet.

It's just too hard to stick with diets that, even though they may be very popular, just don't make sense. For instance, the Paleo diet has some great aspects (avoid processed foods), but also some pointless rules. My daily delicious, healthy, homemade breakfast of steel-cut oats, blueberries, milk, and a spoonful of peanut butter? Absolutely *everything* in it is forbidden on the Paleo diet, except for the blueberries. This makes no sense. And it makes life unnecessarily difficult if you're trying to follow the diet.

Most people can't keep it up. And having, as your main rule, *Eat whatever you like from this list of high-fat, high-protein foods* is both too restrictive, and doesn't help you limit the amount you're eating. And it pushes the idea that carbohydrates are the enemy, when they're not.

I was out with a group of friends a while back. After watching a show, we went out for dinner at a nearby restaurant, MOD Pizza. I go there often, and have my routine meal. The pizzas sold are "personal" size, but they're still huge, and I get a lot of toppings. So, I eat a third of the pizza, and bring the rest home in a box. That's my routine, at this particular restaurant.

A friend of mine, Jill, who was on the Paleo diet couldn't have any pizza (the pizza crust was not Paleo) and ended up having a bowl of salad. A bowl of salad can be a perfectly fine meal if you're trying to lose weight. But this one wasn't. It was huge and full of greasy add-ons such as dressing (sugar-free but very oily) and bacon. It was "Paleo", but definitely had more calories than someone trying to lose weight should have eaten.

The real reason why the low-carb Paleo diet is unworkable for many people is that it has the cause of the obesity epidemic wrong. People are *not* becoming obese because they're eating too many carbs. And people did *not* gain weight over the past few thousand years, as agriculture became more developed, and they started eating more wheat and rice.

No, people gained tremendous amounts of weight in the past 50 or so years, and particularly in the last 30. Obesity was just not a big problem before then.

So, should we look back more than ten thousand years, to pre-agricultural times, to learn to fight obesity? No. Grains and dairy foods are not the problem. And avoiding them with a low-carb Paleo diet is not the solution.

Low-Fat

The low-fat trend has been taken over by low-carb in the last few decades. But back in the 1980s and 1990s, low-fat was huge. It was heavily promoted as a part of US government nutritional policy. Even now, official government nutritional guidelines recommend that we limit fats to 30% or less of calories.

The low-fat trend caused some crazy twists in diet. The popular (mis)conception was that anything low-fat was good. Non-fat or low-fat versions of foods that had been around for thousands of years were thought to be better than the standard versions. So, we had an explosion of low-fat dairy products, like non-fat milk, non-fat yogurt and low-fat cheese. We had low-fat and fat-free cookies. The most famous item, that achieved cult-status and inspired mad rushes at grocery stores, were fat-free (but high sugar) SnackWell's Devil's Food Cookie Cakes.

Here's how the good food/bad food split would look for the low-fat diet:

Low-fat diet	
Good foods	**Bad foods**
Non-fat milk	Cheese
Fruit	Avocado
Vegetables	Sour cream
Non-fat yogurt	Butter
Tuna packed in water	Tuna packed in oil

Low-fat has faded in popularly in the last decade or so, replaced by low-carb. But it remains preserved in government policy. Crazily, it's not possible to find regular, whole milk in schools across the United States. Government school nutrition guidelines require that only low-fat or non-fat milk are allowed. However, very sugary (but non-fat) chocolate milk *is* available.

It's interesting that the low-fat diet recommendations from the US government were first published at the beginning of the obesity epidemic, in the late 1970s. But it's probably a coincidence. Because here's the thing—people did not actually change their diet. They didn't start eating less fat. So, eating less fat could not have caused the obesity epidemic.

Fat is high in calories, it's true. Pure fat (such as vegetable oil) has more than double the calories, by weight, as the same weight of white sugar, or white flour. One gram of vegetable oil has 9 calories, whereas one gram of sugar has 4 calories.

But limiting fats, in particular, is not a good strategy. Humans have a very strong desire to eat rich, fatty foods. That makes it difficult to stick to a plan that very strictly limits the amount of fat you can eat.

White sugar and white flour are bad

White sugar and white flour are *ingredients* in a lot of highly processed, addictive foods that you'd be better off avoiding.

But what happens when people specifically try to avoid white sugar and white flour? Food manufacturers just make ingredient switches in their highly processed foods. For instance, agave nectar or beet syrup instead of sugar. Sometimes it's just a name change, like evaporated cane juice instead of sugar (evaporated cane juice is just sugar). This doesn't make the food healthier.

White sugar is just as "natural" as anything typically called a "natural" sweetener. Natural is really a meaningless word when talking about food products. And having a rule like this leaves the door wide open to all kinds of highly processed, sweetened foods you should be avoiding. Just because they contain "natural" sweeteners instead of white sugar doesn't mean you shouldn't limit them.

And—there's nothing wrong with whole grains. Eating whole grains is often a better choice than refined white flour. But avoiding white flour completely, and only eating 100% whole grains could make life very difficult. And making life very difficult means that it's hard to make this a long-term guideline. For instance, it basically means never eating pizza at a pizzeria, because they rarely have a 100% whole grain crust. Many other restaurants also wouldn't have any options if you followed this rule strictly.

At home, are you never going to use white flour? What if you're baking your own treats, like cookies or a birthday cake? Are you going to use 100% whole wheat flour? It makes baking much more challenging, and changes the taste.

This kind of unnecessary strictness makes life harder than it needs to be. And it doesn't even address the causes of our obesity epidemic. The root cause of the obesity epidemic is the constant, easy availability of highly processed, addictive foods. These foods can be made with whole grains and "natural" sweeteners almost as easily as with white flour and white sugar.

The Health Halo effect

What is the "health halo" effect? It's the way we react when food is labeled with certain terms that we consider "healthy". We then think of the food itself as healthier than it would otherwise be, without the label.

This is a well-studied effect. And the studies consistently show that the labeling and presentation of a food has a big impact on how healthy people think it is, and how much they eat.

One study showed that a particular candy, when labeled as "fruit chew" was perceived as much healthier than the same product, with the same ingredients, when labeled as "candy chew". And another study showed that people who were actively trying to lose weight ate *more* trail mix if it was labeled as a "fitness" snack, with an image of running shoes. When the same product was simply labeled as "trail mix", they ate less.

We're all very susceptible to believing in whatever is considered the latest and greatest food fad. And what's considered healthy has changed dramatically over time.

While visiting some older relatives recently, I ran across a 1956 copy of LIFE magazine. There was an interesting ad for Domino Sugar in it. Here's a few excerpts:

- Domino Sugar is low in calories...high in energy
- Lift up your energy—Hold down your weight the modern way, with Domino Sugar
- Nutritionists know there's no need to go on a sugar-starved diet to keep weight down...in fact, it can actually be harmful to deny yourself the energy of Domino Sugar!

These days, with the epidemic of obesity that we're facing, it sounds crazy to say "it can be harmful to deny yourself the energy of sugar". But some of the health claims that we are surrounded by now will sound just as strange in the future

Low-cholesterol was a huge health-halo buzzword starting in the late 1970s. Some studies appeared to show that having high blood cholesterol caused heart disease. Suddenly, everything that was low-cholesterol was good, and foods that were high in cholesterol were bad.

Eggs became unpopular. Throughout most of history, eggs were considered very healthy, and strengthening. But because low-cholesterol was now "healthy", and eggs have a high level of cholesterol, eggs were suddenly *not* healthy anymore, in the eyes of most people. Egg-white only products became popular, since it's the yolk of the egg that contains the cholesterol.

More recently, studies have shown that cholesterol in the food you eat is *not* closely linked with high blood cholesterol. And that eating a moderate amount of eggs does *not* appear to increase the risk of heart problems. But it takes a long time for the stigma to go away, and many people still believe that eggs should be limited or avoided.

Of the two headlines below, which would be more likely to be remembered, shared and promoted?

Warning—eating eggs shown to cause heart disease!

or

Earlier studies indicating that cholesterol consumption causes heart disease are now found to be flawed.

It's the first one, of course. Humans have a strong tendency to be alert for danger. So, if something is presented as a risk to avoid—that attracts our attention. Something that's less attention-grabbing may not even be noticed.

Currently, "gluten-free" is one of the popular terms used to label foods, and give them an undeserved health halo. Gluten is only a problem for people with Celiac disease, or gluten intolerance—a very small percentage of the population. Still, all kinds of foods are now labeled gluten-free. I just saw some jelly beans at the grocery store, with a prominent "gluten-free" tag in large letters on the front. Of course, jelly beans have *never* had gluten in them. Labeling jelly beans as gluten-free doesn't make them healthier.

***

I went on a field trip to a local grocery store recently, to get a better sense of how many of the foods have some kind of health claims on them. And the answer is—most packaged foods. Here's a sampling of some of the health claims on the packaging.

Kellogg's Raisin Bran Crunch Breakfast Cereal
- 16 grams of whole grain
- Good source of fiber
- Low-fat
- No high-fructose corn syrup
- Heart healthy

(It's still a highly processed, very sugary cereal)

Kashi GOLEAN, Breakfast Cereal, Peanut Butter Crunch
- Excellent source of fiber
- Vegan
- Non-GMO

(Another highly processed, sugary cereal. It uses brown rice syrup as its main sweetener instead of sugar or corn syrup.)

Welch's Berries and Cherries Fruit Snack
- Fruit is the 1st ingredient
- Fat-Free
- Gluten-Free
- 100% vitamin C

(Fruit may be the first ingredient, but it's still candy)

That's it Apple + Pineapple 100% Natural Real Fruit Bar
- High Fiber
- Vegan
- Gluten-Free
- Non-GMO
- Sugar-Free
- No preservatives

118

- Paleo

(There are only two ingredients in this fruit bar—apples and pineapple. But dried fruit is very high in sugar, and there's more sugar in this (51%) than in many candies.)

Annie's Three Cheese Pizza Poppers
- No artificial flavors
- No synthetic colors
- No added nitrites
- 7g of protein per serving
- Made with cheese from cows not treated with rBST+.

(This frozen food is produced by Annie's Homemade, now owned by General Mills. It's not any healthier than any other pizza snacks).

What can we learn from all these examples? Here's some points to think about:

We believe many health claims because we *want* to believe them.

We want to eat the foods we crave most—the high-calorie, hyperpalatable foods. But we also want to feel good about eating them. Often, the more health claims there are on a food package, the better we feel about buying it. This is true even if the claims don't make a lot of sense. For instance, foods like potato chips and jelly beans are being promoted as gluten-free. Well, they never had gluten to begin with. So, they won't be better for you just because they're labeled as gluten-free.

The more health claims there are for a food, the more skeptical you should be.

If you buy some apples or a bag of carrots at the store, what health claims are there on the package? There's nothing. Yet these are very healthy foods. Contrast that to some of the foods mentioned above, with all kinds of health claims.

I would "just say no" to a package of food that has any health claims like these:

- Non-GMO
- No preservatives
- Gluten-Free
- Vegan
- All natural
- Whole grain is the first ingredient
- Paleo friendly

They're trying too hard to convince me, and that makes me skeptical.

Exercise

Another myth is that exercise is the answer to weight loss.

Exercise is great, don't get me wrong. There are many, many benefits to exercise, as I'm sure you hear regularly. And a lack of exercise leads to many health problems, including joint issues, depression, poor muscle tone, etc. People who exercise regularly sleep better, have less anxiety, better memory, and increased energy.

So—what's the problem? The more exercise, the better. We should all exercise very hard in order to lose weight, and to maintain weight loss?

Right?

Wrong. Here's the problem. People give exercise *too* much importance in weight loss. Often, people think that losing weight is half exercise, and half better eating habits. It's not anywhere near that. In fact, you can lose weight without doing any exercise at all. And it's very easy to wipe out the calories you use in a full hour of exercise, with just a few minutes of eating. You can't out-exercise your eating.

✳✳✳

The truth is that working out intensively, and specifically to lose weight, is a bad idea. Reality TV shows like The Biggest Loser featured extreme exercise. The contestants did many, many hours each day of workouts, with specialized equipment and personal trainers. Yes, exercise helped them lose a tremendous amount of weight, along with their very restricted eating plan.

But the answer to the all-important question—whether they were able to *maintain* that weight—is clear. They did *not* maintain their weight loss. Extreme exercise helped them lose the weight, but no lifetime habits were built. They didn't build any routines that worked in regular, daily life. During the filming of the show they had personal trainers working with them, coaching and coaxing them. They had all day to work out, and they didn't have any of the normal demands of life. It's no wonder they weren't able to maintain their weight loss at home. They were in a completely different setting.

Their previous world—of limited food and unlimited exercise—disappeared, and so did their weight loss.

Another problem with extreme exercise for weight loss is that often there's a built-in stopping point. Here's an example. A friend of mine, Randy, got really enthusiastic about running a marathon. I didn't think it was a good idea, because he was obese and already had joint problems. But he did it—prepared for it for more than 5 months, hired a trainer, and did daily training runs and long runs on weekends. He lost a lot of weight. He carefully logged all his routes and times.

So, what's my point here? Running a marathon is good, right? It got him started on a lifetime fitness habit, he lost much of the weight he'd gained over decades, and then kept it off?

Unfortunately, that's not what happened. A week of post-marathon rest turned into a month, and then many months, and now it's been more than a year. He stopped running, and stopped all exercise. During the training period, he weighed himself daily, and lost weight. But after the marathon was over, he had multiple celebration meals. He got out of the habit of daily weigh-ins—he didn't want to, after all those celebration meals. He ended up gaining all his weight back.

This isn't the case with everyone that runs marathons, of course. Many people regularly run marathons, and stay in great shape. It's not the marathon, specifically, that is the problem. When you complete a marathon, that's a great achievement, and something to be proud of.

The problem is if you think of extreme fitness routines as a weight-loss tool. When you cross the finish line of an extreme event like a marathon, it easily becomes an ending, instead of the beginning of a lifetime habit. Gretchen Rubin, in her excellent book on habits called Better Than Before, writes:

A finish line marks a stopping point. Once we stop, we must start over, and starting over is harder than continuing.... The more dramatic the goal, the more decisive the end—and the more effort required to start over.

Most kinds of extreme fitness routines backfire if you count on them for weight loss. For instance, a coworker of mine, Andrew, was determined to get in shape, and lose the extra weight he'd accumulated over the years. Andrew had a friend who was in great shape, with six-pack abs, who went to the gym very early every weekday morning, and worked out for 2 hours. This friend offered to help train him, if he got to the gym every morning at 5:00 am.

Unfortunately, the results were the same as with my friend Randy. Andrew had the satisfaction of telling his friends and coworkers, for about a month or so, that he went to the gym every day at 5 am and worked out for 2 hours. But the workouts were painful. They caused extreme muscle soreness, and injuries.

Andrew's 5:00 am workout was short-lived. It was *not* the beginning of a lifelong exercise habit. It lasted about a month, and then "life got in the way". How could it be otherwise? Andrew had an intense job and three children—he didn't have two hours, every day, to work out.

Is it wrong to experiment with exercise? No, absolutely not. I don't want to give the impression that you shouldn't try to run a marathon, or do extreme exercise routines.

But losing weight and keeping it off in our current food environment is very challenging. It takes work, planning, and figuring what food habits and guidelines work best for *you*. And 95% of losing weight is about what you *eat*, and not how much you *exercise*.

Yes, regular exercise is very healthy. But exercise is the main factor in weight loss and weight maintenance only if you do *extreme* exercise routines. And for most people, extreme exercise routines will not be kept up for a lifetime.

Another piece of advice I've often heard about exercise is "find exercise you really like". And then examples are given like tennis, basketball, etc.

I'm a huge fan of social sports—my sport is pickleball, and I try to play a few times a week. But I know first-hand how tricky the logistics can be. You need to find a place and time that works for many people, and you may need to cancel because of weather. It's great when it works, but it's best not to rely on it for regular exercise.

Instead of an extreme exercise habit, or social sports, go for a walk every day, of 30 minutes or more. Make it brisk if you like, or relaxed. The important thing is that it's convenient, and that you enjoy it. For me, a brisk uphill walk on my treadmill in the basement is easy and pleasant, because I watch my favorite TV shows while I use the treadmill. It's a part of my morning routine, and doesn't take much time.

Exercise doesn't promote weight loss. It seems to help people maintain their weight—active people are less likely to gain or regain weight than inactive people—but it's not associated with weight loss. There are many compelling reasons to exercise, but study after study shows that weight

loss isn't one of them. The way to lose weight is to change
eating habits.
—*Gretchen Rubin, Better Than Before*

Intuitive eating

Intuitive eating is a food and eating philosophy that first became popular in the 1990s, with a book of the same name by Evelyn Tribole. It's based on rejecting "diets", and instead believing in certain principles. It appeals to many people, because one of the main messages is that you have "unconditional permission to eat".

Here's some of the core principles:

Honor Your Hunger Keep your body biologically fed with adequate energy and carbohydrates. Otherwise, you can trigger a primal drive to overeat.

Challenge the Food Police Scream a loud "NO" to thoughts in your head that declare you're "good" for eating minimal calories or "bad" because you ate a piece of chocolate cake.

Make Peace with Food Call a truce, stop the food fight! Give yourself unconditional permission to eat. If you tell yourself that you can't or shouldn't have a particular food, it can lead to intense feelings of deprivation that build into uncontrollable cravings.

Respect Your Body Accept your genetic blueprint. Just as a person with a shoe size of eight would not expect to realistically squeeze into a size six, it is equally as futile (and uncomfortable) to have the same expectation with body size.

It's understandable that people are interested in this style of eating. There's no food that is off-limits. And whatever weight you're at is fine (because it's your "genetic blueprint").

But it's based on thinking that's fundamentally wrong about the causes of obesity. The causes are very, very clear. The majority of people in the United States are overweight or obese now. And it's because we:

- Are surrounded by a variety of cheap, delicious food— food engineered to encourage us to overeat
- Have a biological drive to overeat when delicious food is around

This, alone, will make us gain weight. Unless you've adopted specific guidelines—which I'll go into in the next few chapters— being constantly surrounded by delicious, addictive foods is enough to make us gain dramatic amounts of weight.

It's true for rats, who gain weight very quickly when their plain rat chow is switched to a variety of junk foods (such as pastries, marshmallows, salami, chocolate, sweetened breakfast cereals, etc.). And it's just as true for humans.

Intuitive eating could work, if we only had simple, healthy foods around. If you only rarely encountered hyperpalatable foods, then you could indulge when you came across them, and not gain weight.

But that's not today's world. Today, every day could be a feast day. Our food drive tricks us into thinking that we need to prepare for hunger and famine tomorrow. And in many situations, hunger is not a biological urge that needs to be satisfied—it's just the result of seeing or smelling food that we like.

The Intuitive Eating message of compassion, and not blaming yourself for your weight—that's useful. Blame and shame can get in the way of the work that you need to do for weight management. But the rest of the advice is counterproductive. You'll actually gain weight if you follow it.

Summary

- There are many popular myths about food and nutrition, and what it takes to lose weight. This is because there's no easy "magic bullet" that helps you lose weight, and keep it off.
- There's always a grain of truth in the myths. For instance, exercise does cause weight loss—if everything else stays the same. But over the long term, most people aren't able to exercise enough to keep weight off, without changing their eating habits.
- These myths can distract you. Because they blame obesity on the wrong cause, they offer the wrong fix. For instance, the paleo/low-carb diet says obesity is caused by overeating carbohydrates. Since that's not true, their solution (avoid carbs) doesn't work for most people.

HAZARDS YOU NEED TO AVOID

The worst hazards in our food environment, and some strategies to deal with them

---

In this chapter, I'm going to go through the hazards in today's food environment. These are the food factors that you need to limit, or even avoid completely, in order to lose weight and keep it off.

If you've been keeping track from earlier in this book, you'll recognize these food factors from the section "Food now—tasty, cheap, and everywhere".

They are basically the reasons why we, as a society, have gained so much weight in the past years. The factors that have *caused* many of us to gain so much weight are the very same ones we need to *avoid* to manage our weight.

This makes complete sense. If you have a problem, you need to target the root cause of the problem. But this is often ignored in favor of quick-fix diet solutions that become popular, like low-fat and low-carb. People like an enemy, especially a simplistic one. So, if you can point to one thing (carbohydrates, or fat) as the "enemy", it's very satisfying, and makes a good story.

But the truth is, our current obesity problem is caused by a combination of factors. These factors are:

Our instinctive human desire for a variety of rich, delicious foods

Throughout human history, the people who survived were the ones with a strong drive to eat high-calorie food whenever possible. Those that didn't have this drive often did not survive. Because of this, most people have this same biological drive to eat high-calorie, tempting foods when they're around.

Our current food environment, which delivers exactly what we want—a variety of rich, delicious food

Food has become much more abundant over the past 100 years, and especially over the past few decades. Special occasion treats that were once only enjoyed at feasts or celebrations are now cheap, and available every day. Food scientists develop new, delicious foods constantly, that nobody had even dreamt of 100 years ago.

Also, our culture around food has changed dramatically. Occasions that were not associated with food, decades ago, are now associated with food. For instance, a children's soccer game, or a normal day at the office. Eating in restaurants has become far more common, and making meals at home has become uncommon. Food portions have exploded in size.

These are the factors that have caused us to gain so much weight in the past decades. And in order to lose weight, and maintain a healthy weight, we need to fight them.

We can't fight them directly. For instance, there's no brain surgery or pill to remove our desire for rich, delicious foods. It's hard-wired into our brains, so we're stuck with it. And we also can't change the fact that highly processed, additive, delicious foods surround us.

But there's many other strategies to avoid the hazards below. Learning more about these hazards, and how best to deal with them, is the first step.

Restaurants

The bottom line is, restaurants are dangerous for your weight. Meals eaten in restaurants have more calories than meals eaten at home. And the more often we eat in restaurants, the more we weigh.

This danger is almost impossible to exaggerate. There's a *very* clear relationship between eating restaurant food (including take-out and delivery food), and weight gain.

This has been studied in depth, by multiple researchers, over decades. And it doesn't matter whether the restaurants are fast food places, coffee shops, pizza outlets, family-friendly chains, or gourmet sit-down restaurants. Even those of us who don't eat healthy foods at home will eat even worse in restaurants.

It's *hard* to eat healthy in restaurants. Just recently I traveled with my family to a small town in Oregon, and looked for a place to eat lunch. We chose a restaurant that seemed likely to offer healthier foods. It was advertised as vegetarian, and all the food was made in-house.

I ordered a tomato and cheese sandwich. It was tasty and well served, but huge and dripping with oil. Even though I shared it with my son, it was still far too much, and left me bloated.

So, even with the best intentions, with a better-than-average knowledge of nutrition, and making what seemed like good choices, I ended up with a meal that had far too many calories.

✳✳✳

Why do restaurants serve such large portions? Why do they offer food that's so greasy and unhealthy? Why, even when you order a salad, does it come with all kinds of add-ins such as bacon, blue cheese crumbles, and drenched with oily dressing? Why do they put fresh, crusty bread on the table as soon as you sit down?

The answer is very simple. *That's what consumers want.* If the restaurant doesn't give consumers what they want, they'll go out of business. Large quantities of rich, delicious food are what we, as human beings, desire. That's what customers have told the restaurants we want, with the choices we make. What we generally purchase are the delicious, extravagant meals. The double and triple burgers, with extra fries. The stuffed pizzas with extra cheese. The huge plates—platters, really—of pasta, with rich, succulent sauces.

Restaurants are particularly dangerous because we're eating the food right away. This makes a huge difference in our decision making. It's well-known that when we're making decisions for ourselves in the *future*, we're much more likely to make choices that would be better for the long term. For instance, when we're going grocery shopping, we're buying food to have at home, for future meals. Our tendency is to buy healthier foods.

Compare this to when we're buying food to eat right away—like in a restaurant. The immediate gratification part of our brain takes over—the urge to satisfy our hunger in a big way, now. Our choices are *much* less likely to be healthier.

✳✳✳

Restaurants—particularly fast food restaurants—have been criticized for decades now, for selling unhealthy foods. But there have been many attempts by restaurants to switch to healthier options. It's interesting to learn about the history of these attempts. It tells you a lot about the difference between what we really want, and what we say we want.

The story of the McLean burger, offered by McDonald's for a short while in the early 1990s, is a good example of what generally happens. That era—the 1990s—was the peak of the low-fat trend. And McDonald's was taking a lot of criticism over its generally unhealthy food choices. So, they spent tens of millions of dollars developing the McLean, a low-fat burger. Many more millions were spent on a nationwide advertising campaign, including full-page ads in newspapers, to promote the burger. There were even worries and debates over the supply of low-fat beef. Since there would soon be such a huge demand for the low-fat McLean, what could be done about the coming shortages of low-fat beef?

What happened? Well, there was no need to worry over the supply of low-fat beef. The McLean was soon called the McFlop, and ridiculed on late-night comedy shows.

Initially, there was a burst of sales because of the huge marketing campaign. But most people didn't buy it twice. It was missing much of the fat, and it was also missing much of the flavor of a regular burger.

Most people *said* they wanted healthier options. And criticism of fast food restaurants for their unhealthy foods was intense. But when it came right down to the choices people made, they did *not* buy the McLean at McDonald's. The McLean was quietly taken off the menu a few years after it was introduced.

Customers also did not buy the many healthier options that have been introduced at fast food restaurants over the past few decades. It's been one flop after another. The lower-fat Burger King SatisFries, the Dairy Queen Breeze frozen dessert (made with low-fat yogurt)—all have been discontinued. At Kentucky Fried Chicken, the healthier Kentucky Grilled Chicken appears to be on its way out, and is only offered at a few of their restaurants.

The bottom line is that what people *say* they want (healthy foods in reasonable quantities) is not the same as what they actually choose. When you're hungry, and placing an order at a restaurant, what you choose is usually what your immediate biological urges are screaming for. These are the rich, high-calorie options. Unless you've planned in advance, impulse takes over. You pick the foods that would have been the right choice—if you were living in a time of food shortages and famine.

But you're not. In a time like now, when we're surrounded by food abundance, those choices lead to obesity.

✳✳✳

Here's an interesting story. There's an Applebee's casual restaurant in my neighborhood, and I eat there occasionally. I mostly eat from the Light Eats section, which has their healthier menu options. I was surprised to see, the last time I went there, that the Light Eats section had disappeared entirely. But the healthier menu items were still there. They were just scattered throughout the menu, and much harder to find.

Why is this? Why wouldn't Applebee's make it easier for people to find and pick the healthier choices?

Here's my theory. At Applebee's, there are different types of customers. The good customers are the ones who go there often, and buy a lot. They buy appetizers, drinks, and desserts.

Then there's people like me—not very good customers. I don't go there often, even though it's close to my house. I scan the menu for something healthy, and don't order drinks, appetizers or dessert. I may have eaten an apple or banana before going to the restaurant, so I'm not starving when I get there.

I believe that having a specific section of the menu that was supposed to be "healthy" made their best customers, the customers that went there often, feel uncomfortable. They still chose the foods they wanted—the less healthy foods—but they didn't feel good about it. They were unhappy, being confronted with a supposedly healthy section that they felt they *should* have chosen from.

That's my theory of why the Light Eats section disappeared from the Applebee's menu. People want to eat what they want to eat, and they don't want to feel uncomfortable about it. They don't want to feel like they're making bad choices. This is similar to how some people feel about stepping on the scale. They just don't want to know what their weight is, because they would feel bad if they did.

I spoke to two friends about how the Light Eats section disappeared from the Applebee's menu, and asked both of them why they thought Applebee's did this. One of them—a very slender guy—had no idea. And the other one—overweight, and actively trying to lose weight—immediately came up with the same explanation that I did. He said it probably made the heavier eaters feel uncomfortable. Applebee's best customers felt bad about not ordering from the "light eats" section, so it was dropped.

✳✳✳

What do restaurants want? Obviously, they want to get customers, and make good money. Restaurants need to stay in business, make a profit, and keep up with the competition.

How can they do this? By getting customers to come in, spend lots of money, and come again soon. If restaurants could make good money by encouraging healthy food choices, then we'd find lots of healthy food choices in restaurants.

But that's not the case.

Customers have told restaurants, via their purchasing habits, that they want something else. They want large portions of rich, delicious foods. Customers buy foods that appeal to their immediate urges.

How can you lose weight, while still going to restaurants? How can you maintain your weight loss, in a culture where eating at restaurants is becoming more common than eating at home?

It's tricky. And there may come a time when more restaurants offer a healthy food environment. That will be when customers demand it, and are willing to pay for it. I'm not holding my breath, though. For now, I'm going to give you some strategies on what *you* can do, personally, to make your restaurant visits healthier.

Don't eat at restaurants

Okay, I'm not being completely serious here. But I'm semi-serious.

It's important to realize what a strong connection there is between frequent restaurant meals and obesity. And it's important to understand just how dangerous restaurants are for a healthy weight. That understanding is *fundamental* to learning how to eat out, without gaining weight, and even while losing weight.

Once you accept that, then you're more likely to accept that you need to limit restaurant visits. You're more likely to develop some personal rules and guidelines for when you do go to restaurants.

In modern culture, eating out is far, far more frequent than it was 50 years ago. And in the past 20 years, the percentage of meals that we eat at restaurants has exploded. That's a big part of why we've gained so much weight.

You probably can't or don't want to completely eliminate eating at restaurants. For many of us, restaurants are where we meet friends and family, and socialize. So—if you can't eliminate restaurant meals, then minimize them. Don't make them a regular part of your routine. Don't eat at restaurants for convenience. This includes takeout and delivery meals. Only eat out when it's a social event, or a celebration—try to keep eating out down to once a week, or less. You'll find it much easier to lose weight, and maintain your weight.

Plan restaurant meals ahead of time

As a person that wants to lose weight, or just maintain weight, going into a restaurant is like going into a battlefield. Avoid restaurants if you can. But when you can't avoid them, plan your restaurant visit.

Of course, you can still eat at restaurants, and lose weight, or maintain weight. People do, all the time. But before you go out, check out the restaurant menu online. Look at the calorie counts, when available. Decide what you're going to order. You'll have a much better chance of ordering something reasonable.

Have your own personal restaurant routines

When you do eat out at restaurants, find your favorites, the ones with some healthy options. Decide what your routine meal will be, at these. Having a routine, and having your default choices at particular restaurants, is extremely helpful. There's no decision making, there's no agonizing over choices. Just do what you've done before, if you know it's a good choice for you.

I meet friends at a coffee shop at least a few times every week. If I bought something from their bakery—say a delicious scone, or an almond croissant—I would definitely gain weight. So, I don't do that, ever. My coffee shop routine is to have just my regular drink, which is a cup of tea or coffee. Sometimes I'll add a packet of sugar to it.

Routine is your friend. Variety, and constantly needing to decide whether you're going to get yourself something extra or not, is stressful. Just don't do it.

Fast food can be okay

Fast food has a bad reputation, as a place where only unhealthy food is sold. It's certainly very easy to buy meals at fast food places that are not good for you. Those are what's heavily promoted and marketed. And in general, the customers at fast food restaurants tend to be heavier than average.

However, with some planning, you can buy food that's perfectly healthy at some fast food restaurants. As a matter of fact, I find it much easier to eat a healthy meal at McDonald's than at some other restaurants. At McDonald's I have a routine, a set meal I always eat. But at a restaurant that I don't know, I have no routine. I'm likely to be left with no healthy options.

I was coming home from an overnight hike recently with my friend Patricia, and I suggested that we stop at McDonald's for a burger. Patricia objected, saying McDonald's was too unhealthy. We ended up getting a sandwich at a local deli. Most people would say the sandwich at a local deli would be the healthier option.

But I have a set, routine meal at McDonald's. It's a simple cheeseburger and black coffee. That's what I *always* get. At the deli, I ended up getting a sandwich that had more than twice as many calories as my routine meal at McDonald's. And it automatically came with a side serving of fries. I'll get into personal food rules later on in this book, but this was *before* I had a personal food rule of not eating fried foods. So, I ate most of the fries, even though I wanted to avoid them. For me, it was *really* hard to not eat french fries that were in front of me.

It's up to you. If you have a hard time sticking to healthier choices at fast food restaurants, then you're better off not going to fast food restaurants at all. But sometimes they can be a good option.

Avoid all-you-can-eat restaurants

Buffet restaurants, all-you-can-eat places, or any kind of restaurant where you serve yourself all you want—these places are a hazard for your health. Standard buffet restaurants are becoming less popular, but things like hotel breakfast buffets are more popular than ever.

They have the standard features of restaurants that are dangerous to your weight—lots of variety, and hyperpalatable, rich foods. Plus, they have one additional feature, which is—the more you eat, the better value you get.

If you go to a buffet restaurant and eat a standard sized meal, you have paid a very high price for your meal. If you eat double that, the price will go down dramatically, and you will have gotten a "good value", in terms of calories per dollar spent. If you triple it, you've gotten a crazy good deal—and so on, with no limits, except that of stomach capacity.

Especially if you have a tendency to want to get good value for your money (which is most of us), it's safest to avoid buffet restaurants altogether.

Eat at home before you eat out

If you're going out to eat—especially to a restaurant where you have no routine meal—then you may be better off eating something ahead of time. An apple, a slice of cheese, or something like that. That way, when you arrive, you won't be completely famished. You'll be more likely to order something reasonable, instead of something more extravagant. If you've eaten something before your restaurant meal, then the high-calorie meals won't look quite so appealing.

If you're going out for social reasons, but don't feel like a restaurant meal, then try eating a light meal at home, and just have soup or salad at the restaurant.

My friend Raymond routinely eats a banana and some almonds, and drinks a glass of milk, before heading out to a restaurant. Having something in his stomach helps him make better choices at the restaurant.

Drinks

Soda. 100% Fruit juice. Sweetened coffee drinks such as lattes and Frappuccinos. Smoothies.

In the past 50 years, the consumption of calorie-rich drinks that were *not* milk has increased dramatically. The consumption of regular milk has taken a nose-dive.

High-calorie, sugary drinks such as sodas have a tremendous effect on weight. They go down very easily, and we tend to notice them less because there's no chewing involved. That means we don't eat less because we consume high-calorie drinks. We eat about the same amount, on top of the high-calorie drinks.

So, we know that these drinks are a big source of unnecessary calories. What are some of the potential strategies we can use?

Avoid soda

Soda is a well-known culprit in weight gain. Soda contains lots of sugar or corn syrup, and the serving sizes have gotten larger over the years. Avoiding soda or strictly limiting it is best for most people.

Soda consumption, in the quantities that are common today (the 32-ounce Big Gulp from 7-Eleven, 387 calories) can lead to very quick weight gain. If you drink one 12-ounce can of soda a day, that's 144 calories, or 52,560 calories a year. That's 15 pounds of weight. And the dangerous thing about soda is that we often don't account for them in our mental reckoning on calorie intake. We tend to think of them like water. We tend to think "How much have I eaten today?", instead of "What have I eaten and drunk today?" So, limiting soda is an obvious strategy for losing weight.

The consumption of soda has actually been decreasing in the last few years. People are starting to realize that drinking soda is bad for your health. The problem now is what we're replacing the soda with. Sometimes it's water, which is great. But often people switch to heavily marketed drinks that claim to be healthier, but have just as much sugar, or even more.

Avoid fruit drinks and fruit juices

Fruit juice sounds much healthier to us than soda. And it does occasionally have a few more nutrients than soda. But mostly, it's concentrated sugar with no fiber or other nutrients, just like soda.

Take orange juice. Most people would think that drinking a glass of orange juice is a healthy choice. And it can be a slightly healthier choice than soda (it has some vitamin C, and sometimes fiber). But that same fact—that it's a little bit healthier than soda—makes us drink far too much of it.

Years ago, juice glasses were tiny. They were usually around 4 ounces—half a cup. But now, a medium size orange juice at McDonald's is 12.5 ounces, more than three times that size. And it has 200 calories, more than a can of soda at about 140 calories.

Take a look at this advertising, for a brand of orange juice.

- This premium, non-GMO Project Verified, 100% pure-squeezed pasteurized orange juice is never sweetened, never concentrated and never frozen.
- Uses only simple ingredients that are easily recognizable.

- Oranges are all carefully selected at the peak of ripeness, and no water or preservatives is added to the juice.

It sounds very healthy, right? And so much more convenient than actually eating peeling an orange, and eating it.

But it's this same convenience and the "health halo" effect that makes it so easy to overindulge. To make a "standard" serving size of orange juice (for instance, the medium size orange juice at McDonald's), you'd need 4.5 oranges. Imagine peeling and eating 4.5 oranges. Most people would never do it—but in the form of orange juice, it's easy and convenient. You get all the calories, and none of the effort.

Avoid "healthy" drinks, like smoothies and sweetened teas

The largest soda companies now have all purchased brands that consist of "healthier" drinks. I put healthier in quotes, because although they're promoted as being healthier, they're still highly sugary drinks, and you should avoid them.

For instance, PepsiCo now owns the Naked Juice brand of juices and smoothies. They're not advertised as a healthy *alternative* to soda. Talking about alternatives to soda would imply that soda isn't healthy, which isn't a good idea for a soda company. Still, health claims for these juices and smoothies make up a big part of the advertising.

But many of these juices have the same amount of sugar as the equivalent in soda. Sometimes they even have more. People enjoy them because of our built-in desire for sweet foods, but think they're drinking something healthy because it's fruit juice.

It's not healthy, though. Most fruit juices give you far too much sugar.

Take, for instance, the Green Machine Naked Juice flavored juice blend. It's a very green drink. It looks like somebody took a bunch of spinach, and stuck it in the blender. And this is how it's advertised:

- *Non-GMO Project Verified. No Sugar Added. No Preservatives*
- *Vegan*
- *Boosted with 10 turbo-nutrients including spirulina, alfalfa, broccoli, spinach and kale*

The mention of spirulina, alfalfa, broccoli, spinach and kale— these make people think that this is a healthy drink, like a liquid version of salad. But when you look at the details, you see that the main ingredient is apple juice. The number of calories in one 8-ounce cup is actually more than in the same amount of soda—a lot more, 140 calories vs. 93 calories. And there's no fiber in it *at all*.

I did some research on how much of the "turbo-nutrients" are in a serving. And according to the brand website, it's almost nothing—it totals a little more than 2 grams. That's *grams*, not ounces. One gram is a trivial amount, about the weight of a paper clip.

Most of these 2 grams come from the spirulina, which is a type of algae that has long been used as a health food supplement. And—it has also recently been approved by the FDA as a food coloring...a *blue* food coloring.

Why would you need *blue* food coloring in a drink that's bright *green*? Well, when researching this, I remembered some basic facts about mixing colors. Almost all the main ingredients (apple, mango, pineapple, banana) are yellowish. The ingredients that you'd expect to be green (alfalfa, broccoli, spinach, etc.) add up to a tiny amount—around 2 grams. They're not what's making it green. But if you add blue food coloring to mostly yellowish ingredients, you get green. And people think they're drinking a healthy veggie drink, because of the green color.

Green Machine Naked Juice is a particular misleading food product. But if you dig into it, the advertising is not lying. It's called a flavored fruit juice blend. On the website, the "turbo-nutrients" ingredients are given in exact amounts, measured in milligrams. It's very clear on the nutritional panel that there's a massive amount of sugar in this, and zero fiber.

So, the manufacturer of Green Machine Naked Juice is not directly lying, but they're hoping to mislead. People see a green drink, and they see "spirulina, alfalfa, broccoli, spinach and kale". They understandably think, "I'll just have one of these instead of a salad, it's tastier and more convenient, and just as healthy." And it *is* tastier and more convenient. But it's not a healthy food choice at all.

✳✳✳

Coke is also getting on the bandwagon, and selling drinks that are supposedly healthier. They recently purchased the Honest Tea company, and made it one of their brands. The Honest Tea drinks are sweetened and tea-based. They tend to have less sugar than the drinks based on juice, but some of them are still tremendously sweet, with lots of added sugar.

Honest Tea has a line of drinks designed for kids, called Honest Kids. Here's a note from their website:

In 2013, we removed the organic cane sugar from all Honest Kids varieties. We found a way to deliver the same great taste by sweetening the juice drinks ONLY with fruit juice.

This is another variety of the "health halo" claim. They're implying that this drink is healthier because they removed sugar, and sweetened it with concentrated fruit juice.

But it's not healthier. Concentrated fruit juice is almost all sugar. Your body can't tell the difference.

Avoid artificial sweeteners

What about drinks with artificial sweeteners? Diet Coke, or Splenda in your tea or coffee? Are they a good option? Are they a way to get the sweetness you crave, yet not take in the calories that sugar would give you?

It would seem like it. But there are plenty of problems with artificial sweeteners. The first is that they just don't seem to work the way people think they do. People think—if I drink Diet Coke instead of regular Coke, I'm taking in fewer calories.

Well, that would be true, if everything else stayed the same. But that's not what happens in real life. People think that they're being "good" by having a diet drink. So, they often "reward" themselves by eating something else, like a bag of chips or a pastry.

The Canadian Medical Association Journal published a report in 2017 which looked at 37 studies on artificial sweeteners. And these studies seem to show that artificial sweeteners are linked to weight *gain*, rather than weight loss. People that regularly consumed artificial sweeteners, of all kinds, actually gained weight, and increased their health risks.

Granted, these studies were mostly observational studies. That is, they basically asked study subjects whether or not they regularly consumed drinks with artificial sweeteners. In general, the people that did use artificial sweeteners gained weight, over time.

Another factor that's probably affecting these study results is that people who consume drinks such as artificially sweetened soda—which is a highly processed food—are probably consuming a lot of other highly processed food. And *all* highly processed food is strongly related to weight gain.

The final reason to avoid artificial sweeteners is that they affect your taste for sweetness.

If you start limiting your sugar—you don't drink sweetened drinks (artificial or not), and limit the sugar in your food in general—then normally sweet foods such as a banana or a sweet potato will start to taste sweet.

It's amazing how soon that starts to happen. It just takes a few weeks, and you'll start tasting the sugar in things that previously didn't seem sweet at all. A bowl of unsweetened breakfast cereal with half a banana sliced into it will taste pleasantly sweet.

Avoid sweetened coffee drinks

Here's some advertising from Starbucks on some of their sweetened coffee drinks:

✻✻✻

Mmm, Caramel Brulée Latte, so luxuriously silky and sweet. Sipping one feels like a big, warm hug.

Hot and cool at the same time, the Peppermint Mocha is a boost for your brain and a party for your taste buds.

Have you tried the Toasted White Chocolate Mocha? With subtly caramelized white chocolate sauce it almost tastes like sitting in front of a roaring fire.

***

These drinks sure sound delicious. And they are delicious—they're engineered that way—but they're *very* high-calorie. And right now, they're having an explosion in popularity.

Over the past decade or so, soda drinking has gone down. Sodas are starting to have the feel of a low-class drink. Many people automatically think "Soda = unhealthy". But they don't yet have that association with coffee drinks. Coffee-based drinks—lattes, macchiatos, cappuccinos—still seem sophisticated and classy.

Also, there's been a lot of research recently on the health benefits of coffee. These appear to be pretty well substantiated now—coffee is associated with a lower risk of diabetes, stroke, and cognitive problems like depression and Alzheimer's.

But these health benefits are associated with coffee, plain coffee. They're not associated with the creamy, sugary, high-calorie drinks that we're buying at Starbucks, that have a hint of coffee in them.

These sweetened drinks are highly processed, and designed to be delicious and addictive. They're very high-calorie, and very low nutrition. A standard Starbucks Frappuccino has 430 calories—about a quarter of the daily calorie needs for a typical woman.

It's easy to be misled by the menu offerings in a coffee shop. I met my friend Beth at a Starbucks recently. I had already had a few coffees that day, so I had regular tea instead, unsweetened. Beth had a London Fog tea. Which seems like... a type of tea. But the full name is London Fog Tea Latte, and—no surprise—it was full of added sugar and cream. Delicious, but not something you want to drink if you're trying to lose weight, or maintain your weight loss.

Drink unsweetened tea and coffee instead of sweetened coffee drinks

There's also good news. The good news is that unsweetened drinks, such as coffee and tea, can be very helpful in weight loss. This is because when you're drinking unsweetened drinks, you're *not* drinking sweetened, high-calorie drinks.

And there's another reason that unsweetened drinks can be helpful. How? Because they substitute for unhealthy foods. If you have a mug of black coffee in your hands, it'll be easier for you to avoid the tray of donuts. Or, for instance, at a cocktail party, with trays of appetizers—you'll be more able to ignore them if you have a glass of sparkling water in your hand.

Drink sparkling water and unsweetened iced tea instead of soda and juice

Instead of the sweetened cold drinks, look for the unsweetened ones. There's been an explosion in these types of drinks recently, many different varieties are available. But I would suggest that you consider making your own drinks. It's easy to make a big pitcher of unsweetened iced tea, or lemon water, or cucumber water.

If completely unsweetened cold drinks, such as unsweetened iced tea, taste strange to you, go ahead and add some sugar. But sweeten it *yourself.* That way you're conscious of the amount of sugar in the drink, and you can work your way towards drinking it unsweetened, or with just a small amount of sugar. You *will* get used to lower amounts of sugar, over time.

And remember that *sugar is sugar.* Honey or agave syrup or the latest "healthy" sweetener is no better for you than plain sugar.

Limit alcohol

What about alcohol? I'm going to repeat a few things about alcohol that you probably already know.

- **Alcohol contains a lot of calories.** Alcohol is not one of the standard macronutrients—carbohydrates, fats, or proteins. But it still has calories. The calories in alcohol are higher than pure carbohydrates or pure protein—almost twice as much. They're almost as high as pure fat. And these calories are completely empty of any nutritional value.
- **Alcohol affects your judgment.** The more alcohol you drink, the worse your decision-making will get. Temptations that you might have been able to resist without alcohol (appetizers, a full-size hamburger with fries, dessert) will be much harder to resist.

You don't have to stop drinking entirely to lose weight, or maintain weight loss. But you do need to be conscious of your drinking, and plan it. You need to understand the number of calories that your drink contains.

If you remember, earlier in this book I wrote about how the size of plates and bowls has increased dramatically over the years. Well, wine glasses have undergone an even more massive increase. Glass size increased slowly since the 1700s, and then exploded in the 1990s. According to a study in the British Medical Journal, wine glass capacity increased 7 times in the past 300 years. And of course, larger glasses mean that larger amounts are consumed.

So, you can't just think to yourself, "I drank a glass of wine, that's about 120 calories". You have to make sure that your glass of wine is the size it should be—about 5 ounces. That's just a little more than half a cup.

A friend of mine, Andrew, had lost 40 pounds over a year. He did this by weighing himself daily, on top of slowly making changes in his diet. But then he hit a plateau. He still had 20 pounds he wanted to lose, but wasn't able to get there.

Andrew figured out that part of the problem was the beer he loved, and drank regularly. It was one of the real pleasures of his life, and he didn't want to give it up. But drinking a full bottle was too much. He did some research online to find techniques for keeping the beer in good shape, without finishing a whole bottle. Once he had that technique working, he happily drank just part of a bottle, and kept the rest to drink later.

Processed, hyperpalatable foods

Remember the "hyperpalatable foods", from the chapter "The History of Obesity"? Hyperpalatable, highly processed, pre-made foods are the ones that grab us, the ones that we have a hard time saying "no" to. These are the foods that are addictive for some people. Some people have the same relationship to their favorite hyperpalatable foods as heroin addicts do, to heroin. Just being around those foods sets off a craving that is hard to fight.

✳✳✳

Until recently, food processing had two goals. One was to make the food more digestible. For instance, whole wheat kernels, before they're ground into flour, are not very digestible. Our bodies have a hard time getting calories out of them. But, ground up into flour, and then baked into bread, it's filling and satisfying.

The other reason for processing was to make the food last longer. Drying grapes to make raisins, making cheese from milk—all these are ways of preserving food. These types of food processing were developed because the original food (grapes, milk) would spoil in just days without processing. Raisins and cheese, though, can last for months or years.

But now, things are different. The new food products that are coming out are *not* ways to make food more digestible. And they're *not* new ways of preserving fresh foods.

Instead, they make foods tastier. The new food products are more fun, and more convenient. Thousands of new processed food products come out every year—either entirely new products, or new varieties of old products. For instance, the Lemon Oreo cookies are a very successful twist on the regular chocolate Oreo cookie. And the new candy bar Hershey's Cookie Layer Crunch (with flavors such as Caramel and Vanilla Creme) is a more processed, more exciting version of the standard Hershey's milk chocolate bar.

These foods have been engineered by dozens of food scientists and chemists. They have been tested and tweaked to appeal as much as possible to consumers. Teams of marketing consultants decide on the colors, slogans, and other advertising that will help make the new product a hit.

Here's a short sampling of some of the most popular highly processed foods around.

Highly processed foods

- Kellogg's Raisin Bran Crunch breakfast cereal
- Organic Peanut Butter and Cocoa Balls breakfast cereal by Whole Foods 365
- Clif Bar Cool Mint Chocolate protein bar
- Chocolate Peanut Butter Flavor protein bar by Luna
- Blueberry Acai Probiotic Juice by GoodBelly
- Honest Kids Organic Super Fruit Punch
- Ben & Jerry's Strawberry Cheesecake Ice Cream
- Cranberry Bliss Bar by Starbucks
- Cheetos Crunchy Cheese Flavored Snacks
- Trader Joe's Inner Peas Baked Green Pea Snack
- Sourdough King Burger from Burger King
- Bear Claw Pretzel Bites with Beer Cheese from Red Robin

What are some of the characteristics of all these highly processed foods? Here's a few:

- They taste great. People love them, and have a hard time eating just a little.
- They're "new" foods. Most have been around for less than 50 years.

- They're extremely convenient—you can eat them without any work at all. Food goes straight from the package to the mouth.
- They're processed so that they can last a very long time. Many of the protein bars, breakfast cereals, and sweets would taste just the same in six months as they do now.
- There's a huge variety of them. Most of the foods you see in supermarkets are highly processed foods like these.

Next come the foods that have some processing, but are not highly engineered foods developed in food laboratories. Some of these foods (flour, bread, raisins, cheese) have been around for thousands of years, and some of them (canned foods, frozen foods) are more recent.

Foods with some additional processing

Wheat flour
Bread
Dried fruits, like raisins and dried apples
Yogurt
Cheese
Vegetable oils
Canned vegetables
Canned fruit
Pasta
Frozen vegetables
Frozen fruits
Jam
Butter

Peanut butter

Mayonnaise

Sugar

Unprocessed foods

And then these foods are mostly unprocessed. Very little, other than packaging and storage, was done to these foods.

Honey

Eggs

Meat

Milk

Apples

Blueberries

Kiwis

...and all other fruits

Lettuce

Squash

Sweet potatoes

...and all other vegetables

Wheat

Oatmeal

Rice

...and all other grains

Lentils

Peanuts

Walnuts

...and all other nuts and legumes

Reasonable people can disagree on the level of processing allowed to consider a food "unprocessed". For instance, I have milk in the list, but almost all milk is now heat-treated with pasteurization to kill bacteria. And all fruits, vegetables, and grains available in stores have been through thousands of years of breeding, to make them larger, or sweeter, or whatever trait the farmers want.

The level of processing that a food goes through can vary widely. For instance, here's the blueberry, from least to very highly processed:

- Wild blueberry, eaten immediately (completely unprocessed)
- Fresh blueberries, purchased at a grocery store (the blueberry has gone through many years of selective breeding, and was grown on a large-scale farm)
- Blueberry jam (jam, as it exists today, has been around since the 1800s)
- Frozen blueberries, purchased at a grocery store (another processing step—today's freezing process was developed in the 1920s)
- Blueberry Pomegranate Smoothie with Yogurt from McDonald's (a highly engineered and processed food, developed in a laboratory with food scientists, and extensive consumer testing)

Here's an interesting thing about the last two categories— unprocessed foods, and foods with some additional processing. The list of foods is *short*. And, more importantly, *it's not growing*.

Think about that for a moment. Yogurt has been around for thousands of years. And people have been eating cheese since the time of ancient Egypt. But almost all *new* food products are highly processed, hyperpalatable foods.

For instance, take the example of Go-Gurt Portable Low-Fat Yogurt by Yoplait. It's a sweetened low-fat yogurt product, developed in the late 1980s. It was inspired by sample squeeze tubes of shampoo that you find in hotels. The most dramatic feature of this product is how convenient it is. It's designed to be slurped, single-handedly, from a tube. No spoon necessary. No need to sit down to eat it.

Or, take some of the most popular breakfast cereals that were introduced in 2017.

- Apple Cinnamon Toast Crunch
- Nature's Path Dark Chocolate & Peanut Butter Love Crunch Cereal
- Nutter Butter Cereal
- Donut Shop Pink Donut Cereal
- Chocolate Peanut Butter Cheerios

All of these new foods are very highly processed, and very delicious.

✳✳✳

Are all highly processed foods evil? Are they bad for you? If you're looking for a simple answer, then I'll say this:

The more you're able to avoid highly processed food, the easier it will be for you to lose weight and keep it off.

Because these foods are so addictive and convenient, for many people it's easier to avoid them completely. They're so hard to stop eating, that you may be better off if you never start.

You would likely lose weight if you ate no highly processed foods, and you'd avoid a lot of unhealthy foods. And this kind of rule may work for some people. But if you don't want to, or can't completely avoid highly processed foods, try to limit them as much as possible. Or, you can avoid certain types of highly processed foods (for instance, salty snacks).

Highly processed foods are definitely not bad in the sense that they're toxic in the short term. They're not, of course. People eat massive quantities of highly processed food all the time, and don't die.

But do these people, the ones that are eating mostly highly processed foods, gain large amounts of weight? Do they die sooner than they otherwise would have? And are more people suffering from disease and disability because of eating too much highly processed foods?

The answer is yes, yes, and yes.

So, we need to understand the whole issue better.

These foods are not toxic, and they're not poisonous. But generally, the more highly processed foods you eat, the worse off you are. They're *strongly* associated with obesity. This is a tricky situation, if you're trying to create rules and guidelines for yourself.

Cigarettes are easy—they're very unhealthy, and you can live just fine without them. They may be difficult to give up, but there's no question that you should definitely stop smoking. People aren't putting cigarettes in front of you constantly, and there's no cultural pressure to smoke.

But food is different. You need to eat. And you have a very strong biological urge to eat large amounts of tasty, delicious foods—like highly processed, hyperpalatable foods. Given a choice between a fresh apple and a delicious glazed donut, most people would pick the donut. Our brains are designed to crave rich, calorie dense foods, so we pick them when we have a choice.

Here's a few more things we can say about highly processed foods

- They're cheap, convenient, and abundant. They surround you constantly
- They taste far better than simple, unprocessed foods
- They're heavily marketed, with all kinds of hype
- If you eat them in small quantities, they could be fine
- It's very hard to eat only small quantities

Could you live a healthy life, eating mostly highly processed foods? Could you lose weight, and then stay at the right weight, without limiting highly processed foods?

Some people might be able to. If you were able to control the number of calories you ate, while eating mostly highly processed foods, then they probably wouldn't do you much harm.

But right there is the problem. Most people have a hard time eating limited amounts of these foods. They're very hard to stop eating. These are foods that are *engineered* to be addictive, and hyperpalatable.

And most people in the United States live this way now, eating mostly highly processed foods. The consumption of highly processed foods is going up, and up, and up. And so is the rate of obesity.

✳✳✳

What are some guidelines and advice for living in a world where highly processed foods are all around you? Most people are eating highly processed food constantly. What should *you* do?

I give more ideas later on in the book on food rules you can develop for yourself. And below are a few potential guidelines that are specific to highly processed foods. But importantly—what works for you will be highly personal. You'll need to figure what is best for *you*, and implement that in a way that fits your lifestyle.

Understand the dangers of highly processed foods

The first step in deciding how you want to limit your consumption of highly processed foods, is understanding just how dangerous they are.

If you have a clear understanding of the link between highly processed foods and obesity, you'll understand that you need to limit them somehow. And without this, you're unlikely to make and stick to changes. You just won't have the motivation, unless you clearly understand how vulnerable you are to weight gain from eating highly processed foods.

You may want to review the section about highly processed foods in the chapter "The History of Obesity". That section has details on the addictiveness of most highly processed foods, and the links between eating these foods, and weight gain.

Avoid highly processed foods

The best advice here is to just *avoid highly processed foods*. Avoid the foods that are ready-to-eat and pre-made, where you just open the package and dig in. Salty snacks like potato chips and crackers, energy and protein bars, sweetened breakfast cereal. Lots of frozen food is fine (such as simple frozen fruit and vegetables), but highly processed frozen foods should be avoided.

I do *not* suggest that you avoid the foods from the list of "Foods with some additional processing". These are the foods that have some processing, but are not completely premade and ready-to-eat. So, foods such as cheese, bread, canned vegetables, frozen fruits and vegetables, jam, sugar, etc. Usually these foods are fine. And *avoiding* all these foods entirely would involve a huge increase in the time you spend preparing food, or a big change in what you eat.

Also—these are foods that have been around for a long time. In some cases—like bread and cheese—thousands of years. They're not what's causing the increase in obesity. What's causing it is the fact that we're eating so much highly processed, addictive foods, and so many more meals at restaurants. And that's what we need to limit.

Remember earlier, in the suggestions for how to deal with restaurant meals, I suggested avoiding restaurants entirely? Well, the same applies to highly processed foods. I *suggest* that you avoid them totally. But realistically—you probably won't be willing or able to do this. So, what you need to do is two things:

- Understand that highly processed foods are addictive and dangerous if you don't limit them
- Figure how best *you* can limit highly processed foods— which *personal rules* you'd be happy to live with

Be skeptical of food advice that demonizes one ingredient

One ingredient that has gotten a lot of attention recently, as an awful food that you should never eat, is high-fructose corn syrup. It's supposed to be spectacularly bad for you, as well as a marker for highly processed foods that you should avoid.

Why is this misleading? High-fructose corn syrup has been a bad-guy ingredient for some time now. But it's just another form of sugar. It's cheaper to manufacture than regular sugar. This is why so many manufacturers switched to it when it first became available in the 1970s and 1980s.

What else happened in the 1970s and 1980s? Yes—the rate of obesity in the United States also began to skyrocket. So, in people's minds, the rising obesity rate was linked to—and maybe caused by—this new sweetener.

This wasn't the case, of course. High fructose corn syrup was an *ingredient* in many of the highly processed foods that were coming onto the market. But it wasn't the high fructose corn syrup that was causing the obesity epidemic. It was the fact that people began eating large quantities of convenient, highly processed, addictive foods.

Demonizing high fructose corn syrup, or ingredients like it—this leaves you vulnerable to health hype marketing. You can be misled by simple ingredient switches. These ingredient switches don't affect how healthy a food is.

For instance, since high fructose corn syrup became unpopular, some food manufacturers have begun replacing it with products like brown rice syrup. But brown rice syrup is a type of sugar. It's is no better for you than high fructose corn syrup.

Instead of thinking, "This must be healthy because it has no high fructose corn syrup", you'd be better off being very skeptical about highly processed foods marketed with health claims. Avoiding the latest, trendy "bad" food ingredient, whether it's high fructose corn syrup, gluten, sugar, carbs, dairy, or whatever—won't be helpful in the long term. We didn't gain weight because we ate these foods. And we won't lose weight by avoiding them.

Be skeptical of manipulated ingredient lists

There's another common way that food manufacturers manipulate their ingredient list, without actually making the food product healthier. A few years back, articles started showing up in popular magazines, recommending that people buy breakfast cereal where "whole grain is the first ingredient". Shortly after that, guess what started happening? Whole grain became the first ingredient in many breakfast cereals. Often a prominent label was put on the front of the package, saying "Whole grain is the first ingredient".

But the fact that whole grain is the first ingredient doesn't mean much. If the first ingredient is whole grain oats, but the next three ingredients are different types of sugar—say, brown rice syrup, organic evaporated cane juice, and agave nectar—then you still have a product with lots of added sugar.

Imagine there's a new brand of breakfast cereal. Let's say that these are the percentages, by weight, for the first 4 ingredients in this new cereal:

Ingredient	Percentage of total
Whole grain oats	18%
Brown rice syrup	17%
Organic evaporated cane juice	16%
Agave nectar	15%

So, the amount of whole grain in this breakfast cereal is 18%, but the amount of sugar (every ingredient after the whole grain oats) is a total of 48%. It's almost half sugar. But the product could still be advertised as "whole grain is the first ingredient".

Here's a real-life example. The protein bar by Clif Bar (vanilla almond flavor), has the following 4 items at the top of the ingredient list, in order:

- Soy protein isolate
- Beet syrup
- Organic brown rice syrup
- Organic cane sugar

Then there's a total of 29 other ingredients, some of them vitamins, totaling 33 ingredients. None of these ingredients are inherently bad, but if you're trying to avoid too much sugar, and take a quick look at the ingredient list, you'd think it's okay. The first ingredient is *not* sugar, or a type of sugar. However, the next three ingredients *are* different types of sugar.

This protein bar has almost as much sugar as two Oreo cookies. By using three different ingredients (beet syrup, organic brown rice syrup, organic cane sugar) as sweeteners, instead of just using one, they can manipulate the ingredient list. They avoid having sugar first on the list.

Most ingredient lists aren't going to be as misleading as this example. But still, you need to be aware of this issue.

The problem is that we really *want* to believe that our favorite tasty highly processed foods are healthy choices. Food manufacturers want to help us in this illusion. So, we turn over the package, take a quick look at the ingredients, and—not seeing sugar as the first ingredient, or not seeing high fructose corn syrup— decide it's healthy.

But it's probably not.

Be skeptical of food products that claim they have a simple list of ingredients

The list of ingredients on most foods today is long and complex. Many of the ingredients are items you can't find anywhere in a grocery store. And you'll find many food products with 20, 30, or even more ingredients (such as the protein bar above, with 33 ingredients).

As a reaction to these long ingredient lists, this kind of advice has started popping up:

Avoid food products that contain more than five ingredients.

While I think it's a good idea to look at the ingredients, it's also another way that you can be duped. A rule like this can lead to a whole set of foods being avoided, that would be otherwise totally fine. For instance, whole wheat bread bought in a store will usually contain whole wheat flour, yeast, salt, sugar or honey, some seeds and other grains, and some type of oil. That's more than five ingredients. I sometimes make whole wheat bread at home, and my standard recipe has 8 ingredients (I add sunflower seeds and a few other grains).

So, if you follow this "5 ingredients only" rule you may rule out foods that would be completely fine. And, on the other side, you could leave the door wide open to foods that you should mostly avoid.

Because here's what's happening. Food companies have noticed that many consumers are unhappy with long, complex ingredient lists. As a response, they're starting to produce food that has a limited number of ingredients. But many of these foods are no healthier than foods with long lists of complex ingredients.

For instance, Häagen-Dazs has a line of ice creams called Five. These all contain only five ingredients. The coffee ice cream contains cream, milk, sugar, egg yolks, and coffee.

And Frito-Lay's now has a line called Simply. The Simply Lay's Sea Salted Potato chips contain only three ingredients—potatoes, sunflower oil, and salt.

***

Lärabar is a manufacturer of energy bars, and they were one of the first to promote a limited ingredient list. The company was built around the concept of selling energy bars with a short list of simple ingredients. For instance, their Cherry Pie bar contains just dates, almonds, and cherries. Their other fruit and nut bars contain between 2 (Cashew Cookie, just cashews and dates) and 9 ingredients (Pumpkin Pie flavor, with dates, almonds, walnuts, raisins, dried pineapple, coconut, carrots, cinnamon, and coconut oil).

These foods, with a short list of limited ingredients—are they actually better for you? Would avoiding foods that have more than a certain number of ingredients (say 5) be a useful rule?

I doubt it. Why should it? Just because a highly processed, hyperpalatable food contains less than 5 ingredients doesn't make it any less addictive than one with 20 ingredients. It doesn't make you less likely to overindulge in it. It could actually make you *more* likely to overindulge, because you could think to yourself, "It only has 5 simple ingredients, it must be healthy".

✻✻✻

In general, be skeptical of *any* health claim on the label of a food product. If a food manufacturer claims that a product is healthier because it's gluten-free, or has no high fructose corn syrup, or has a limited set of only 5 ingredients—don't buy it.

Usually, as soon as a health claim for certain foods is made, and becomes popular, it's used in advertising. This is not because food companies have some evil master plan to feed us unhealthy foods. It's because these are the things consumers want:

- Tasty foods. We love delicious foods, we love variety and novelty.
- A clear conscience. We want to eat these tasty foods, but we want to feel good about it. We don't want to feel guilty that we're eating junk food.

Food companies are giving us what we want. They're helping us feel good about eating these highly processed foods, by marketing them as "No high fructose corn syrup", "Certified GMO free" or "Only 5 simple ingredients".

But they're not really better for us.

Summary

Restaurants: It's very hard to not gain weight if you frequently eat at restaurants. Restaurants offer the foods that they do (large portions of high-calorie foods) because that's what people buy. Some strategies for dealing with restaurants are:

- Eat at restaurants less often.
- Plan restaurant meals ahead of time.
- Have restaurant routines—healthier meals you always order.
- Fast food can be okay, if you order the right thing.
- Avoid buffet and "all-you-can-eat" restaurants.
- Eat something at home before you go out.

Drinks are another potential food hazard. It's easy to overlook how many calories they have, because we don't notice them in the same way we notice food. Some strategies for limiting your drink calories are:

- Avoid soda.
- Avoid fruit drinks and juices.
- Avoid supposedly "healthy" drinks like smoothies and sweetened teas.
- Avoid artificial sweeteners.
- Drink unsweetened tea and coffee instead of sweetened coffee drinks.
- Drink sparkling water and unsweetened iced tea instead of soda and juice.
- Limit alcohol.

Highly processed foods are convenient, delicious—and addictive, for many people. Figuring out strategies to limit them is extremely important, because they're one of the main reasons for our weight gain. Some potential strategies are:

- Understand the dangers of highly processed foods.
- Avoid highly processed foods as much as possible.
- Don't be fooled by health claims—be skeptical of food advice that demonizes one ingredient, manipulated ingredient lists, and food products that claim they have a simple list of ingredients.

FOOD RULES: HOW THEY CAN WORK FOR YOU

What food rules are, and how they help you make better choices every day, without stress

There's one rule that's critical, and the foundation of weight management. That is, of course, weighing yourself daily. That's the one core routine that you can't skip. It's the basis of awareness of your weight and how your eating habits affect your weight. The scale is your honest, blunt friend, and it doesn't lie.

Without the weigh-in habit, it's easy to gain weight without even realizing it. A friend told me that she gained 40 pounds in just three years—but those three years were ones when she *never* stepped on the scale.

Did she gain weight because she didn't step on the scale? Or did she not step on the scale, because she knew she was gaining weight? There's no clear answer, but we do know that there's a very close link between weight gain, and not weighing yourself.

✳✳✳

But enough of that. You're weighing yourself daily now. You're convinced that it's the right thing to do, and you plan to keep it up for a lifetime. Maybe you already had the habit of weighing yourself every day, and what you've read here has just reinforced that habit.

What comes next?

The obvious answer is to eat less. The reason people are overweight and obese is because they eat more calories than they burn. But—specifically how to eat less? What do you eat, and what do you not eat? What rules and guidelines should you follow, to help you eat fewer calories?

Maybe you're one of those lucky people for whom daily weighing is enough to lose weight. Just the awareness of your weight, and the desire to lose some weight, may be enough to get you to eat less. Perhaps you can make the necessary decisions (half a sandwich instead of a whole, skipping the french fries) and not need to think about it very much.

Many people are not that lucky. Or maybe our bodies have changed. Perhaps just weighing yourself was enough to not gain weight when you were younger, but things have changed as you've gotten older.

This is how it was for me. Even with daily weighing, I had a tendency to gain weight—weight that was hard to lose. Most of us need to *consciously* change how we eat. We need to plan what to do differently, and decide on rules and guidelines for ourselves.

In today's world, which constantly surrounds us with delicious, tempting, even addictive foods, we need to draw the line somewhere. If we just eat whatever foods are easily available, we will gain weight. We need to figure out where the line is, between the foods we eat and the foods we don't eat.

And this is what your personal food rules will do for you. By setting them up, you define for yourself where you will draw the line. You develop, to your own satisfaction, the rules that will help you lose weight, and maintain that weight loss in today's world.

But before we get into the details of food rules, let's talk about moderation and abstinence.

Moderation and Abstinence

You can abstain from a lot of things. You can abstain from sex, alcohol, or any type of food. Vegetarians abstain from eating meat. Vegans abstain from eating any animal product, including dairy and eggs.

My eyes were first opened to the potential benefits of abstinence by Gretchen Rubin's book *Better Than Before: What I Learned About Making and Breaking Habits*. She divides people into two types—Abstainers and Moderators. When trying to avoid something like french fries, Abstainers do better when avoiding it completely, while Moderators are fine with having a little.

Abstinence, in the sense of completely avoiding certain foods, has a bad reputation. Recently I was talking to a friend of mine, Ryan who's actively trying to lose weight. We were talking about moderation and abstinence. He had an *immediate* negative reaction to the word abstinence, and we chatted about that for a while.

It turned out that what he really didn't like was the idea of someone else laying down the law, and giving him a set of rules. He never wanted to hear something like, "You may never eat ice cream again". Or whatever the forbidden food was.

Well, I'm not going to tell you that. *You* are the one that decides on your food rules—I'm just giving you some suggestions to consider. But I will present an alternative viewpoint on moderation and abstinence. Here it is:

Abstinence can be much, much easier than moderation.

A lot of mainstream advice on diet and eating habits advise moderation. You practice moderation by changing your habits a *little* bit. Instead of eating a large piece of cake, eat a small piece. Instead of eating three Oreo cookies, eat one. At the movie theater, instead of buying the large bucket of popcorn, buy a smaller bucket.

According to this advice, no food should be "forbidden". Just eat it in moderation. Making a food forbidden—abstaining from it completely—will cause you to crave it. Craving it will cause you to binge on it, and things go downhill from there.

That's the theory, anyway. This might be great advice, for certain people. But you've probably heard it many, many times before. And it probably hasn't helped you one bit. It sure didn't help me.

Why is advice on moderation often useless? Why is it that trying to *moderate* what you eat can be harder than *complete abstinence* from a particular food? Here's some of the reasons that moderation can fail miserably.

Moderation can be stressful and mentally exhausting

Let's take, for example, Samantha. She's at a fast food restaurant with her family for lunch. Samantha is trying to limit the number of french fries she eats. She knows it's a bad idea for her to eat more than just a few, so that's her goal. But inside her head, the constant back-and-forth between the "eat more fries" side and the "stop eating fries" side continues throughout the whole meal. Here's what the debate in her head looks like:

Eat more fries

- I'm extra hungry, I haven't had anything to eat all morning.
- If I don't eat them, they'll go to waste, and waste is bad.
- I took a really long walk this morning—I deserve more food.

Stop eating fries

- I shouldn't eat too many fries, they're not healthy.
- I'm never going to lose weight if I eat fries like this.
- Even though I took a long walk, fries have so many calories that I'd have to walk even more.

This can be stressful. In yesterday's world, it would have made sense to eat as many fries as you could. You have powerful biological drives pushing you to do exactly that. In today's world, where foods like french fries are always available and inexpensive, you need to monitor and limit how much you eat. Always trying to restrain yourself and figuring out when to stop eating can be stressful.

Moderation is tricky to figure out

Take the previous example, with Samantha and the french fries. All the reasons that Samantha came up with for herself, both on the "eat more fries" side and the "stop eating fries" side? *Every single one* is completely valid. So—theoretically, it *does* make sense to eat more fries if you took a really long walk. And they *will* go to waste, if she doesn't eat them. And so on.

Here's the problem, though. If your rule is moderation, the number of fries you can eat ranges between 1 and the whole serving. Say you have a large portion of fries in front of you, from McDonald's. It's more than 500 calories for the whole thing, and about 100 fries. So—at every point between the first french fry, and the 100th french fry, you have a micro-decision to make. Should I stop eating fries, or keep eating fries?

Obviously, you're not going to go through the pros and cons of each side, for each bite you take. But for most people, moderation is very difficult because it's so unclear *when* you should stop. And theoretically, in this example with the fries, it could be at any point, between 1 and 100 fries.

✱✱✱

What would abstinence look like in this situation? For instance, say you came up with a personal food rule for french fries—that you would avoid them completely. Nobody imposed it on you. Nobody forced you to do it, you just decided to stop eating fries for a month, to see what it was like.

The first benefit is that you have a clear, black and white rule. It's often called a "bright-line" rule. There's no wiggle room, nothing left for interpretation. You just don't eat fries.

The next benefit is that—this is a good rule in terms of nutrition. By avoiding french fries, you're avoiding a food that has no real nutritional value. And avoiding them would lower the number of calories you're consuming. You don't need the calories, and would be better off without them.

The third benefit is that this rule (*No french fries*) is not difficult, in terms of eating in the real world. Some rules can be very hard to follow. For instance, if you had a strict rule like "No white flour", that would be tough. Many foods that would be otherwise fairly healthy, would be off the list. And in many restaurants, you'd be restricted to eating salads.

But *No French Fries* is not hard. French fries are always a side dish. If they normally come with your meal at a restaurant, you can make a substitution. The rule doesn't add a lot of stress or hassle to your life.

It's important to know that abstinence is a workable option, and can be the best choice for you. Food rules don't always need to involve completely abstaining from certain foods. But you should understand this, because it's often overlooked:

*It may be much easier to **never** eat some foods, instead of trying to eat just a little.*

You don't want to develop food rules that help you lose weight and keep it off—but cause stress, and constant focus on what you're eating. That's nobody's idea of a good life.

What you want is to figure out the food rules and guidelines that will help you lose weight and keep it off, happily and without too much stress. And considering a food rule that involves abstinence, instead of moderation, can help with this.

So, here are three main benefits of having a personal rule to avoid french fries

- It's a clear, black-and-white rule. There's no confusion about what's okay, and what's not.
- By avoiding french fries, you're not missing out on a healthy food, and you're reducing calories.
- It's easy to follow—you can still go to any restaurant and have a meal.

The first benefit, having a clear rule, is important. It saves a lot of stress. But notice that the next two benefits come from the fact that it's a *good* rule. It works in terms of nutrition, it's not difficult to live with, and it reduces the number of calories you take in. This may seem obvious, but it's important that the food rules you make are *good* rules.

Owning your food rules and guidelines

You have brains in your head,
You have feet in your shoes,
You can steer yourself any direction you choose.
You're on your own,
And you know what you know,
And YOU are the one who'll decide where to go.

Who develops your food rules? You do. That's the way it has to be, so that you can keep following them, for a lifetime.

Ownership of the whole weight loss process is one of the most important factors in success. The book *Keeping It Off* by Robert H. Colvin is an older one, published in 1985. But Dr. Colvin did something that few researchers have done, either before or since. He did an exhaustive search, via radio advertisements and newspaper ads, for people who had lost large amounts of weight, and kept it off for many years. He and his team surveyed these people, trying to get at the common core of their success.

What were some of his findings? The most important one was that most of the people who successfully kept the weight off did it *on their own*. They usually were *not* successful in groups, or with weight loss counselors. These situations put them in the role of a patient, following rules given by somebody else.

No, they were successful when they took responsibility, and made their own rules. They tweaked and experimented with their food habits. Some of their strategies worked, some didn't.

Of course, the principles of weight loss are the same for everybody—you need to take in fewer calories than you use. Once you're just trying to maintain the same weight, you need to take in about the same number of calories that you're using up.

Is there only one way to do this? Of course not. With your daily weigh-in to give you feedback about what works and what doesn't, you can and should experiment. You can try different food rules, routines, and guidelines. Over time, you'll figure out which ones work best for you.

Food rules are the rules that you make *for yourself*, about what you eat and how you eat. They might be rules like "I don't eat fried foods", or "I don't eat after 8 PM". You don't break these rules, unless for exceptions that you decide are okay, like "I don't eat fried foods, except when I fry the food myself".

They're explicitly *not* just taking a food plan developed by someone else, with the good foods/bad foods that someone else has defined, and adopting those 100 percent.

In the "Food rules to consider" section, I give you a set of food rules that may (or may not) work for you. You need to look at them with a critical eye. You need to decide which rules make sense for you—which ones you could be happy with, and potentially keep up for a lifetime.

Do they *need* to be for a lifetime? Not at the beginning, when you're trying them out. You need to figure out what works for you, as an individual, for losing and maintaining weight. You'll need to modify your rules and eating habits based on what helps you manage your weight well. You need to tweak them to make sure you're happy with them, in the long term. This is what will make weight loss possible. This is what will help you keep the weight off.

But once you have a set of food rules that work for you—then yes, you follow them for a lifetime. You have to consider them lifetime rules, because you want to manage your weight for a lifetime.

✷✷✷

The basic principles of losing weight are very simple. You need to lower the calories you take in on a daily basis. But *how* you lower calories—there's infinite variations in how you can do this. And of course, your scale will be your honest, blunt friend. It will tell you if what you're doing is working, or not. It will tell you whether you need to adjust your habits, or tweak your rules.

Food rules are decisions, made in batches. You decide ahead of time what your rule is. This way, you don't have to make decisions in the heat of the moment, when you're faced with temptation.

Maybe you've decided ahead of time: *I don't eat fried foods.* You've committed to sticking with it for at least a month to see how it works.

Then, when you're eating dinner with friends, and someone orders a tempting order of fried onion rings, "for the table", you know you won't have any. You don't need to even think about it, because *you've already decided.*

What are some features of a good food rule?

Following the rule helps you reduce your calories.

The food rule I mentioned above—no french fries—passes this test. By not eating french fries, especially if you previously ate them often, you could really reduce the number of calories you're eating.

I was poking around on the web recently for thoughts on food habits and rules, and found one guy's thoughts on setting food rules. I found it unusual, to say the least. His idea was that you should only make food rules that are easy to follow, and avoid foods you don't really like. In his case, it was...candy corn. He didn't particularly like it, so it was on his "avoid for life" list.

Now don't get me wrong, I'm all for food rules that are not too hard to follow. But this one—to avoid a type of candy that you don't like, and rarely eat—how useful is that? How many calories will you avoid by following this rule?

Many common food rules don't pass this test, of helping you reduce your calories. For instance, *Don't eat refined sugar*. Sure, it has the *potential* to reduce the number of calories you take in. But many people just switch their sugar intake to a more "natural" type of sugar (brown rice syrup, fruit juice concentrate, honey, etc.). Instead of buying the standard, mass-market sweets (regular Oreo cookies, for instance), you buy the "natural" version of that same product. And that version can be just as highly processed, just as addictive, just as sweet, and just as unhealthy.

The rule addresses the root of the problem—why we're all gaining weight.

The root cause of the obesity epidemic is that we're constantly surrounded by convenient, high-calorie, delicious, highly processed foods. Because we have a strong drive to eat, just being surrounded by these foods is enough to make us gain weight.

If your food rule doesn't target a highly processed, high-calorie food, or somehow make it easier to avoid the temptations of these foods, then it's useless. It may even work against you.

For instance, a friend of mine, Cynthia, was recently on a very expensive commercial diet plan. It involved going in for weekly weigh-ins at their center (they forbid weighing yourself at home), and pre-packaged meals. Dinner each day was an "on-your-own" meal that you cooked yourself, but with a *very* strict list of foods to avoid. On this list of "bad" foods were:

182

- Onions
- Sweet potatoes
- Tomatoes
- Corn
- Green peas
- Carrots
- Many other vegetables
- All fruits except for some berries

So, any fruit or vegetable with even a tiny amount of natural sugar was forbidden.

Even if this were an easy rule to follow—would it result in weight loss? No, because it doesn't address the root cause of obesity.

Yes, there were other foods on the "bad" list that would be good to avoid, like pastries, cookies, cake, etc. But overall, it was extremely strict, and eliminated many healthy foods. And it didn't work—my friend wasn't able to stick with it. She lost about 20 pounds on the program. But once it was over, she stopped going into the weight-loss center for her weekly weigh-ins, and gained all the weight back. The program was just too restrictive.

The food rule doesn't make life too difficult.

There are lots of food rules that make your daily routine difficult. Some of these more difficult rules, like eating vegan, are a part of your identity. You *are* a vegan, so you eat only vegan foods. You're okay with the fact that it's difficult.

But in general, the more difficult your food rule is, the less likely you'll stick with it. The food rules you set up for yourself should be as easy as possible to follow—while still being useful for reducing your calories.

I recently reviewed a diet book with some food rules that would have been *really* hard to follow. Basically, all these foods were on the "bad" list:

- Any food that comes in a box
- Any food that needs to be defrosted
- Any food that comes in a can

The *goal* was that you should eat only fresh foods, such as fresh poultry and meat, and fresh fruits and vegetables. But the *reality* is that this type of rule would make life far more difficult. And—it wouldn't necessarily make the foods I eat any healthier.

For instance, I eat oatmeal with blueberries for breakfast every morning. The blueberries are frozen, and frozen foods are not allowed, so I'd have to switch to fresh blueberries. Using fresh blueberries would also mean I'd have to shop multiple times a week, because they don't keep very long. Plus, they're very expensive. And the oatmeal itself comes in a box—that's not allowed either.

So, you need to think about how realistic a potential food rule is. And if your food rule makes it impossible to find a restaurant where you could eat with friends, that may make life too difficult.

The best food rules actually make life *easier* for you, rather than more difficult. How does this work? Let's take, for instance, the "no french fries" rule. I've been following this for some time, and it makes my life easier.

Here's how. Before I had this rule, I never just completely indulged, and ate as many french fries as I wanted to. I ate fries, but while I did, I often felt conflicted, and had the stressful thought in my head, "I should probably stop eating fries soon." And I would often feel bad about eating "too many" fries, even though "too many" wasn't defined.

Now I find it so much easier to just not eat french fries. If I never start, I never need to decide when to stop.

The food rule is crystal clear.

This is the beauty of having a rule. It's not a wishy-washy guideline that you follow most of the time, but break when you feel like it. It's a black and white thing. You've either followed the rule, or not. There's no debate, and there's no slippery slope.

If you had a rule like "Eat fried foods in moderate quantities", then there would be a slippery slope—what is a moderate quantity? That would be a useless rule.

But suppose you adopt the rule "No fried foods". You're at a restaurant, eating a burger. You didn't order fries. The people you're eating with did order fries, and they're eating them, but you're not. So—you followed the rule.

Most people won't have this food rule

Be prepared for other people to think you're a little strange to have *any* food rules for yourself.

Here's the facts. More than 71% of people in the United States are overweight or obese. This is not because they're flawed, or lazy, or have no willpower. It's because we're now living in a food environment that surrounds us with convenient, delicious, addictive foods.

One hundred years ago, we were not yet living in this type of food environment. Most people were also not overweight or obese. But now we are—because of our food environment.

Most people don't have food rules for themselves. Throughout human history, it hasn't been necessary. In earlier times, food was much harder to produce, and was limited because of that. There were frequent famines, and periods of hunger. Only kings and queens had a chance to become overweight.

But it's very different now. It's a new world, in terms of the amount and type of food around. And our behavior has not adjusted.

Most people won't have the food rules you design for yourself. They won't have *any* food rules. And they will probably think that your food rules are weird. For instance, say you have a rule that, before you start eating dinner at a restaurant, you get a take-out container and put some of your food in it. Lots of people will think this is a strange habit.

***

Most people who are thin *do* have food rules for themselves. They won't necessarily call them food rules. But they'll probably have some kind of personal policies that help them limit how much they eat. It could be something like "I never eat fast food", or "I never eat after 7 PM."

A friend of mine, Sara, is slender. She told me about a comment that one of her friends made recently—a friend who had gained a large amount of weight over the decades. The friend commented to Sara, "You're so lucky, you can eat whatever you want and not gain weight."

Sara didn't say anything, but inside she was thinking, "No, that's not true". The truth is, Sara *does* have food rules and policies that she follows. And it's these that have helped her maintain her weight.

She doesn't have some kind of magic metabolism. If she just ate whatever she liked, she'd gain weight.

What's normal, today, is to be overweight or obese. And "normal" behavior leads in that direction. So—be abnormal. Have food rules that some people think are weird.

Food rules should make the food you want to limit *less convenient*.

Inconvenience is much more important than we think. For instance, if your gym is inconvenient to get to, you're far less likely to exercise. If it's not on your daily commute, you probably won't go often. If your dental floss is in an inconvenient spot—in the back of a drawer, say—you're much less likely to use it.

Our eating habits are one of the areas where inconvenience and convenience have a strong effect. There's been a lot of research on this. For instance, people eat a lot of candy if it's in a bowl right on their table. They eat much less if it's in a bowl that's one table away from them. When the bowl is covered with a glass lid, they're also less likely to reach in. And when the see-through glass bowl is switched out for an opaque bowl, they were even less likely to eat the candy.

Making the foods you want to avoid *less convenient* is a great way of limiting the amount you eat you eat. So, what are some food rules that make some foods *less convenient*? One is to just not buy it—don't have it at home. Or you could actually make it *impossible* to buy the food (don't bring money with you, if you're likely to be tempted by foods you don't want to eat).

Making food less convenient, is, of course, just another way of changing our food environment. In general, our food environment constantly surrounds us with highly processed, addictive, convenient foods. Anything that we can do to make this type of food less convenient is a good thing.

Some people need to take drastic steps, to make their trigger foods less convenient. Below is a comment from an online weight-loss forum, by a man who became very obese from eating fast food and junk food from convenience stores:

> *The only way I managed to finally break this binge-eating cycle was to give all my money, credit cards, etc., to my wife as a temporary measure. I allowed myself zero spending at all. For six whole months, I carried no cash or cards on me, and my wife did all the shopping and made all the other household purchases.*

This was a drastic step to take, but it worked for him. He lost—and kept off—a huge amount of weight.

The rules need to be *your* rules.

If you accept a list of food rules, handed down by a doctor, a weight-loss guru, or a book, then you're accepting that other people are dictating something really important—how you eat. This may work for you.

Or, more likely, it will not. The people promoting these food rules don't understand your lifestyle. They're not familiar with your living situation. Eating is very personal—how can they know what's best for you?

The basic principles of weight loss and weight maintenance are always going to be the same. Eat fewer calories than your body uses, and you'll lose weight. Eat about the same number of calories, and you'll stay the same weight. When you eat more calories than you need, you'll gain weight. This is basic science, and there's no debate about it.

But when you're trying to lose weight, the *way* that you accomplish this—limiting your calories—is extremely personal. I would even say—the *more* personal, the better.

For instance, suppose a big problem for you is free cakes, cookies and pastries at work. Many offices and workplaces have tempting food constantly available for birthday celebrations, meetings, and work lunches. And if they're around, you eat them.

So, you decide on a food rule: *I don't eat free food at work.*

This focuses on *your* specific issue, with a solution that *you* would be happy with. You're much more likely to stick to a rule like this. Rules and eating plans handed to you by someone else won't be as useful.

Also, if it's your rule, you're less likely to "cheat"—in other words, break the rule. Instead of "cheating", you make an adjustment to the rule, to fit your lifestyle.

Food rules can have exceptions

You may be the type of person that just doesn't like to hear the word *never* in a food rule, as in *I will never eat french fries again.* That may be a deal-breaker for you.

If this is you, then try tweaking the rule to include an exception. For instance, instead of *I will never eat french fries*, consider a rule like these:

No french fries, unless I make them myself
French fries or hamburger, not both
French fries only on Sunday

Any food rule you create can be made acceptable, even if you just don't like the idea of saying "never". Just throw in an exception to your rule.

The exceptions that work best are the ones that involve some effort on your part, like making it yourself. That makes it less convenient, and less of an impulse decision, but you still get to indulge when you're willing to put in the effort.

I have this as an exception for all my food rules—if I make it myself, it's fine. So, for french fries—if I ever wanted to get out the potatoes, slice them up, and fry them myself, then that's perfectly okay. I haven't yet wanted to do that, but if I did, it would be fine. If I don't want the fries enough to put some work into them, then I don't really want them.

I mentioned above, as a potential food rule: *French fries only on Sunday*. But in general, I'm not a fan of food rules that have a once-a-week exception. Especially for highly tempting, addictive foods— indulging once every week can keep you hooked. And following the rule can be much harder than it needs to be, if you always need to think of what day of the week it is.

But keeping the exception much less frequent (say, on your birthday) or making sure that the exception involves effort (you have to make it yourself) can make it a better rule.

A few more exception ideas are:

Except when I finished [insert achievement here]

When you achieve something (for instance, ran a marathon, started a new job, passed an exam) is a good time for an exception to your food rule. You don't run into occasions like this very often, so it's a reasonable time to make a planned exception to your food rule.

No exceptions

Especially when you're starting out, you may feel that adding exceptions could jeopardize a food rule that works well. And that's fine too.

Summary

- The world has changed, and in today's world of delicious, tempting, addictive foods, we need to draw the line somewhere. Food rules help you create a bright line between foods you eat, and foods you don't eat.
- Many people promote "Moderation" (no food is ever completely forbidden) as a weight-loss strategy. But for many people, moderation can be very hard.
- Abstinence—never eating certain foods—may be easier than moderation. By reducing choices, abstinence can reduce food cravings and obsessions.
- Your food rules are *yours*. You decide on the personalized rules that work best for you.
- A good food rule will:
  - Help you reduce the calories you're taking in.
  - Target one of the main causes of obesity— restaurant food, drinks, and highly processed foods.
  - Not make your life too difficult.
  - Be crystal clear. You either followed the rule, or not.
- Exceptions to food rules are fine. You decide whether you need them, and what they are.

FOOD RULES TO CONSIDER

---

*Here's some potential food rules.
Decide which ones will
work for you*

Below is an assortment of food rules that have been helpful to many people for losing weight, and keeping it off. Some of them should work for you.

I suggest that you put a check mark next to the food rules that you think might work for you. These food rules are the ones that would both reduce the number of calories you take in, and not be unreasonably hard for you to follow. Also—these rules should inspire you to come up with some potential food rules on your own.

This list is definitely not a complete list of potential food rules. Just think of it as a source of ideas, and a jumping-off point for figuring out your own rules. And of course, none of them are mandatory.

And I know I've repeated this often, but it's worth saying it again. The test for whether a particular food rule or set of rules works for you is the scale. Are you able to lose weight and keep it off? This is what matters, in the end. Your daily weigh-in habit will let you know which food rules are effective.

Say you've decided on a set of rules, and have been following them for a while. If you're trying to lose weight and the number on the scale isn't moving down, then you need to tweak them. You need to adjust your rules, so they work for you.

I recently saw a comment online in a book review, written by a man who had adopted a set of food rules outlined in the book that he was reviewing. And in his book review, he complained:

After a month following these rules, I stepped on the scale, and learned that I had actually gained weight!

I have two comments here. Number one—good for him, that he was trying to change his eating habits. But number two—waiting a month, then stepping on the scale to figure out if an eating plan is working for you—that's *not* a good idea.

You need to be weighing yourself *every day*. If you haven't lost some weight—it doesn't have to be much—by the end of a few weeks, it's time to adjust. Change your food rules.

Don't eat french fries

We went through this one in detail before. Avoiding french fries completely may be a relatively easy way to restrict the number of calories you're taking in, while not being too difficult.

For me, fries are a food that I find very difficult to eat "moderately". Once I've started, I don't want to stop eating them. It's *so much easier* for me to just not start.

There might be some foods that I would regret missing out on, if I never indulged in them. But french fries are not on this list. I would never leave a restaurant, thinking, "I really wish I had ordered some of their fries."

Don't eat any fried foods

This rule takes the "don't eat french fries" rule and goes a step further. The "don't eat french fries" rule is great—but it really only helps you at restaurants. French fries are a big source of low-quality, zero-nutrition calories at restaurants.

But french fries are just one of the many fried foods that contribute zero to our nutrition, but far too much to our calorie intake. Take chips and other fried, salty snacks. For instance:

- Tortilla chips
- Potato chips
- Corn chips

And I'm not just talking just about the mass-market chips. I'm also talking about the fancier versions, the more gourmet versions, that are often promoted as a healthier option to regular chips. These fried snacks were some of my favorites, but they were making me gain weight. So, I don't eat them, and it doesn't bother me. For me, they're similar to french fries—eating "just a few" is very hard, but not eating *any* is much easier.

Don't eat any salty, highly processed snacks (fried, or otherwise)

This takes the rule even further. Now, on top of anything fried, we're also avoiding crackers like Cheese-Its. We're avoiding supposedly healthier "baked, not fried" version of foods like potato chips.

Many food manufacturers are switching to baking their salty snack foods instead of frying them. Here's the thing, though—it doesn't really affect how healthy the food is. And it's just as addictive.

I looked at some Cheez-It Baked Crackers recently, and compared them to standard potato chips. They're just a tiny bit lower in calories than the potato chips.

Since I love salty snack food, I would have a very hard time with this rule, if I didn't make exceptions. For me, making the snack food myself is the right exception. I often make delicious homemade popcorn at home, using butter or coconut oil, and salt. The fact that I actually have to *make* it, and it takes a little bit of work, cuts down on how much I eat. But it's not difficult. I make it from scratch, and it takes about 5 minutes.

If I'm ever tempted by salty, high-calorie highly processed foods, I tell myself, "I'll make some popcorn when I get home." This makes the food rule easy to follow. And you're not limited to popcorn—all kinds of simple recipes for salty snack foods (homemade crackers, microwave potato chips) are available online. Once you've made them a few times, you'll realize how easy they are.

These salty snack foods surround us. They're in every vending machine. They are ever-present and ever-tempting. If these are a problem for you, avoiding them completely, and only eating salty snacks that you make yourself can make a *big* difference in your calorie intake.

No sweets unless I made them myself

The desire for sweetness, for sugar, is a very basic one. It's deeply rooted in our biology, because sugar (in the form of glucose) is needed for brain function, and energy. Our ancestors who craved sugar, and ate as much of it as possible—these are the ones who survived, and had children.

Sugar can make us happy. Babies are sometimes given sugar water to relieve pain from medical procedures. A favorite trick of photographers is giving babies a little bit of sugar water, to make them smile.

The bottom line is, we have a *very* strong biological drive to eat sweet things. And this is a problem, nowadays. With modern food technologies, sugar is cheap and very easily available. It's just like many other foods that are causing us to gain weight.

And we're not eating just plain sugar, of course. We're eating sugar in the most tempting, delicious forms. We're eating sweet baked treats such as croissants, cupcakes, and cookies; all kinds of candies and candy bars; and all varieties of frozen treats like ice cream. New sweet treats are invented every day by food manufacturers.

Sugar is not evil or toxic. But sugar consumption, at the level it's at now, is far, far higher than it should be. I'm absolutely not going to tell you that you should never eat any sweets or sugar. That's not workable, except for a very small number of people. But I will suggest that you limit added sugar.

Extreme limits on sugar and sweeteners are very difficult for most people, over the long term. A friend of mine who was on an extremely low-carb and zero sugar diet dropped it after a few months. Why? She hated never having anything sweet.

So, what's a reasonable, sustainable way to limit sugar?

I suggest this rule:

No sweets unless I made them myself

If you're able to stop purchasing sweet treats, and instead make your own, then a few things will happen. The first is that **sweets will be less convenient**. A food rule that prevents you from buying these types of treats will change your food environment—there will be fewer sweets around. And this is what you want. You want the highly processed, high-calorie, addictive sweetened foods to not be around.

Your food rule will prevent you from stocking up on them, in bulk, at the grocery store. You won't have big Costco-sized packages of sweet treats in your pantry. Instead of getting a muffin or a cookie whenever you get a coffee at the coffee shop, you'll skip it. If you really want something sweet, you'll make it later at home.

Another bonus of having a food rule like this is—**you'll expand your skills in the kitchen**. Instead of always buying whatever the latest tempting sweet treat is, you'll learn to satisfy your sweet tooth by yourself, by cooking with basic ingredients. If you're not really interested in learning to cook, then maybe just some very simple recipes to mix a few ingredients together, like cocoa, sugar, and milk for homemade chocolate milk. There's a whole world of recipes

198

available online, for every level of cooking skill. Learning new skills is empowering. You do not need to buy sweets. You can make them yourself, and you'll become a more competent person when you do.

Another effect of this rule is...you can still eat sweets! You won't eat nearly as many sweet treats as most people do, but you could still have something sweet every day. There's no need to feel deprived.

For some people, there's a potential trap in this rule. Some people *love* to bake, and wouldn't mind baking up batches of different kinds of cookies or cakes every day.

So, you need to know yourself, and know what your tendencies are. Maybe you'd need another food rule, like, "I only bake sweets once a week", or "My maximum calories for sweet treats is 100 a day". Or, limit the amount of sugar for home baking that you buy, something like, "I only buy 5 pounds of sugar every month."

My personal exception to this rule is that when friends make some kind of sweet baked treat, I indulge. For instance, at a recent Thanksgiving, a friend made 3 different types of homemade pie. I had a small piece of each one. That's an easy exception to make, because it's such an infrequent thing.

Don't buy any foods with added sugar

This is a variation on the rule "Make your own sweets". But with this rule, we're defining "sweets" more broadly. Instead of sweets being the standard sweet treat (cookies, cake, ice cream, donuts, etc.), we define it as anything with added sugar.

And that means about 99% of breakfast cereals, and almost all yogurts should be avoided. Most granola bars. Most canned fruits. Lots of milk substitutes (almond milk, rice milk).

This does *not* mean that you can't add your own sugar. Feel free to buy the no-added-sugar version of foods—like plain yogurt—and add a spoonful of sugar or jam to it. But make sure you're adding it yourself, and not letting the food manufacturer add it for you.

This rule can get a little tricky, because so many foods do have added sugar to them. Even most peanut butter has added sugar. It's fine to have a few exceptions, you'll just have to figure out what they are. For me, peanut butter with some added sugar is fine.

I make my own junk food

Junk food can be defined in different ways. Let's say that you define junk food as all salty snacks (including chips, crackers, seasoned nuts, and fries) and all sweet snacks (including baked goods, candy, and frozen treats). I suggest that you include protein bars, energy bars, and granola bars in the category of "junk food". These can be especially dangerous because they're often marketed as "healthier" snacks, which tricks us into overeating.

If you follow this rule, it means that you are now going to either stop eating junk food, or make these foods yourself. This will reduce the number of empty calories you're eating. It makes the foods you want to avoid *less convenient*. And it helps you avoid one of the major causes of obesity, which is purchased junk food. In general, people aren't gaining weight because they're making their own cookies, crackers, and other treats at home. No, they're gaining weight because this type of junk food is so convenient and cheap to buy.

But—you're not completely denying yourself junk food. You're free to eat the salty or sweet treats you desire, it's just that you need to put some work into them. They won't be completely identical to the packaged junk foods you can buy, but they can be close.

Eat one type of chocolate

There are some treats that I'm not willing to avoid for a lifetime. And I also don't want to make them myself.

Chocolate, in this food rule, is a stand-in for whatever food that you don't want to stop eating, don't want to buy, but you want to limit. For you, it may be something like ice cream.

I don't want to abstain from chocolate just because it's a highly processed candy. And I'm also not willing to actually make the chocolate myself. I know it's not impossible, and I've seen some recipes for homemade chocolate online. But it seems like a fussy process, and I just don't want to do it.

So—where does that leave me? Here's how the rule works for me.

I buy and eat only one type of chocolate, and have about one piece a day. Sometimes two.

I buy the Dove Promises brand, the dark chocolate variety. They come in small pieces (about 40 calories each), and each individual candy has an inspiring quote on the inside of the wrapper, which is fun to read.

This brand has been very successful, and many different varieties are now available (almond, peanut butter, mint, caramel, cookie crisp, and so on).

If I did a taste test of each of the varieties, I'm sure there I would find another one that I like better than the dark chocolate—probably the caramel variety.

But the point is, I don't need to eat the variety that would be my absolute favorite. It's better for me to have a variety that I like, but isn't overwhelmingly delicious and "crave-worthy". My goal is not to have a treat that's the high point of my day. My goal is to have a treat that works well for me, over the long term.

I don't need or want variety. In fact, having lots of variety would make me want to eat more.

I feel no deprivation. I enjoy my chocolate. But having a rule like this is an easy way to limit my consumption of chocolate and candy. I do it by saying no to anything that is not *this one specific* type of chocolate.

✳✳✳

Say your food is ice cream. You want to avoid buying pre-made sweet treats, in general, and are happy with that rule. But you don't want to avoid ice cream for a lifetime, and also don't want to make your own.

So, you need to figure out what kind of food rule could work in your situation. In the case of ice cream. I suggest a simple flavor, like plain vanilla or plain chocolate, not something with a lot of add-ins. That way you could add whatever toppings you want for flavor and variety (chopped peanuts, strawberry slices, etc.).

Decide on a serving size that works for you. And then buy that (just enough, without stocking up) once a month, or once a week, or on whatever schedule works for you.

With a rule like this, you're limiting your consumption of ice cream, but you're not abstaining completely. You're having it on a schedule that's closer to what would have been common, about 100 years ago. Back then, ice cream was a special event, only made for celebrations.

The bottom line is, you can still have whatever treat you love. You just need to figure out the right food rule, so that you can enjoy it within reasonable limits.

Don't eat free food

Food is often used as a tool. People who are trying to sell you something, like a timeshare—they'll offer a huge assortment of delectable food, to get you feeling good. And after you've eaten their food, you feel like you need to listen to their pitch.

Or people who are trying to sell you financial services—they will often invite you to a free dinner at a fancy restaurant, to make you feel obligated to them. If you just ate the free dinner and then left, you'd feel like a cad.

Just recently, I was at a community meeting. At the back of the meeting room were trays of giant muffins and cookies from Costco. I looked them up online—it turns out that just one of these muffins has about 690 calories! That's almost half the calories that an average-sized woman needs, in an entire day.

At this particular community meeting, they weren't trying to sell anything. But it's become a cultural norm, now. At almost any event, there will be food. Often there will be huge quantities of highly processed, unhealthy foods.

This has become very common in offices and other workplaces. As a feel-good treat, sweets are brought in. Some pastries, or the latest fancy cupcakes from the trendy shop nearby. At an office that I used to work at, every Wednesday was donut day, with dozens of donuts brought in, all different varieties. It was always stressful to resist them or try to limit them by trying to eat just half a donut. Today, if I were in the same situation, I would just tell myself *I don't eat free food*.

Just for fun recently, we went to an RV dealership. They had hot, delectable pulled pork sandwiches there, as an enticement to stay longer, and talk to the salespeople.

It's possible for this type of thing to just be a fun, enjoyable treat in the average person's week. But it's more likely to be a big factor in weight gain. We're so often surrounded by highly processed, highly tempting, high-calorie junk foods, *that are free.* And this can be the kiss of death to weight loss and weight maintenance. I have a tendency to want to take advantage of freebies, so these types of situations were very tough for me.

If you're often in these kinds of situations, and you're constantly stressing over how much of the free food to eat and when to stop, I suggest a blunt rule.

Don't eat free food.

If you didn't pay for it, you don't eat it. It's simple, and straightforward. This is a great rule for when you're at the office, and all the types of situations mentioned above. All those bowls of candy on people's desks? You didn't buy them, so don't eat them. Free candy bars at a convention you're going to? Skip them.

In the past few years, many hotels have started to have complimentary, freshly-baked cookies at their front desk. They take advantage of a weak moment, when you're just arriving at the hotel. Perhaps you've just come off a long plane trip, and are tired. They want you to have good feelings towards their brand, and food is a cheap way to do that. So, they offer you a delicious, warm cookie.

But if you haven't made a conscious decision to buy the food, and haven't spent your own money on it—then don't eat it. The people offering the free food don't care if you gain weight. They don't care if you have a hard time losing weight. It's not their problem.

But it is *your* problem. So just don't eat free food.

Don't eat highly processed foods

This rule is very forceful and blunt. And if you decide to adopt it, some of the other rules would become unnecessary. You wouldn't need a separate rule to avoid highly processed sweet treats, and another to avoid highly processed salty snacks.

In a previous chapter of this book, there's a section with examples of highly processed foods, foods with some additional processing, and mostly unprocessed foods. This is where you'll see the types of foods you need to avoid, and which foods are fine.

And of course, you are creating your *own personal food rule*. So, you would draw the line wherever you think is best. And you would make whatever exceptions that you need, in order to make this rule work well for you.

Highly processed foods make up a large part of most people's diet. And these highly processed foods are exactly what I'm suggesting that you don't eat, with this rule. So, if you choose to follow it, you'd be eating very differently from most people. This is not a bad thing—it's a good thing, since the majority of people have very poor eating habits.

But I would suggest taking it slowly. Let it simmer for a while, before you decide that it's actually what you want to do.

Personally, I don't strictly follow this rule. I *mostly* avoid highly-processed foods, but I make some exceptions. I have so many exceptions that I couldn't really say that I don't eat highly processed foods. But even if you choose to just *mostly* avoid these foods, and have a lot of exceptions, you'll be better off. You'll be able to avoid a lot of calories, while not stressing endlessly over which individual foods should be on your "approved" list, or not.

The default exception I would make here is—if you make it yourself, it's fine. If you bake the cookies (or cake, or pastry) yourself, and it's not causing a problem with your weight, then enjoy it.

Highly processed convenience foods are not inherently bad. They're not poison, and the companies selling them are not evil.

But drawing the line here, and completely avoiding highly processed food, can be very useful. This rule will help you avoid many of the factors that are making our society obese.

If this kind of food—highly processed, extremely convenient, and deliciously tempting—were only available occasionally, then it wouldn't be a problem. But it's not. It's available, and tempting us, all the time and everywhere. And new varieties of these addictive, tempting foods are developed every day.

That's why making a rule like this can be a great idea. Don't force yourself to constantly make decisions about when, and how much highly processed food to eat. Just say no to all of it.

Never eat food from a vending machine

If you adopt the previous rule (Don't eat highly processed foods), then you wouldn't consider buying food from a vending machine. All the food in vending machines is highly processed, so they would be off your list.

However, it may be that you don't want to completely avoid highly processed foods. But perhaps eating from vending machines is contributing to your weight problem. In that case, this may be a food rule you want to follow.

If you decide to adopt this rule, I would suggest that you have some healthy foods with you—say, a piece of fruit, or some nuts— when you'd normally feel the urge to buy something from a vending machine.

If you're really tempted by vending machines, and if you have a hard time with the rule, then here's an idea. Don't just make a rule. Make it impossible.

What does it mean, to make it impossible to get food from the vending machine? Well, you have to pay for the vending machine food, of course. So, make it impossible to do that. Say it only accepts only $1 or $5 dollar bills. Then you need to make sure you don't have $1 and $5 dollar bills in your wallet. If the vending machine accepts credit cards, then empty the credit cards from your wallet.

You wouldn't necessarily want to do something like this forever. But if you have a serious vending machine habit that you want to break, consider this technique.

Forget about willpower. Willpower can be weak, especially when confronting a long-standing habit. Make it *impossible* to do something you don't want to do—in this case, buying junk food from a vending machine

Don't eat your trigger foods

I have to go zero tolerance on nuts, chips and chocolate. If I eat one, I eat the entire bag.
—From the online Reddit LoseIt forum

For some people, certain foods trigger overeating. And once the door is opened to that food—once that first bite is taken—they can't stop.

For these people, the answer is straightforward, though not easy. *Just don't take the first bite.* That's what gets you in trouble. That's what starts you down a path that you have a hard time getting off.

This is the absolute opposite of moderation. It's saying—this food is so dangerously tempting that I can't eat it *at all*. And considering the similarities between food addiction and drug addiction, it's not surprising that some people need to do this.

These foods may be your absolute favorites. But if you really do have problems controlling yourself when you eat them, maybe you need to stop eating them.

Don't eat after dinner

Snacking in the evening can be a major source of unhealthy, unneeded calories. For many people, evening is when their desire for food kicks into high gear. The fridge and pantry are nearby, and tempting.

Out of control, unplanned eating in the evening can be a real difficulty for some people. It can be caused by a combination of these factors:

- Easily available junk food
- Habit
- Not eating enough during the day
- Sitting on the couch most of the evening

It's not that eating in the evening is somehow metabolically different. A calorie eaten in the evening is the same as a calorie eaten in the morning. But since evening eating is less controlled, it can get out of hand more easily.

How do you get back control? One way is to just make a personal food rule—no snacking after dinner. And there's lots of variations and exceptions you could try. For instance:

- Only eat fresh fruit after dinner.
- Only eat unshelled peanuts after dinner (or something similar, that takes effort to eat).
- Only eat 200 calories or less after dinner.

Eating 200 calories or less after dinner *does* involve calorie counting. But it's so limited that it could work for you.

Evening eating is an area where many people have serious issues. Once an evening eating habit is well-established, it can be tough to break it. One very valuable technique is to *not keep the tempting food available in your home*. Don't keep the junk food that you find irresistible in your house.

Eat a maximum of one restaurant meal a week

Remember the section earlier, about the food hazards to avoid? Restaurants, of course, were one of them. If you're like most people and eat out a lot, developing some personal food rules for restaurants will be important.

These rules will vary, depending on your preferences and life situation. And setting a strict once a week limit on your restaurant meals is one way of doing this.

If you're not at home for lunch, this means bringing your lunch most days. If you haven't been in the habit of bringing lunch from home, this could be a big step. You may want to work up to it, instead of immediately trying to bring every lunch from home, every day.

Before starting your meal at a restaurant, put some of it in a take-out container

This is a great restaurant rule, that allows you to visit restaurants that you'd otherwise need to avoid. Many restaurants give such enormous servings that even when you're able to share a meal with a partner, it's still far too much. Even if you just ate half the meal, you'd be overeating by a tremendous amount.

If you don't want to completely avoid these restaurants, here's one potential rule for you. When you order your meal, ask that a take-out container be brought, at the same time as your meal. When the meal comes, put some of it in the container. This should happen before you start eating. Only keep the amount you think is a reasonable serving on the plate.

If you're still hungry after eating your meal, wait ten or fifteen minutes. It takes a surprisingly long time to feel full, especially if you eat quickly.

I eat quickly (it's a bad habit I'm trying to improve), and just recently I finished a meal at a Thai restaurant nearby. Before I started eating this meal, I put much of the meal in a take-out container, and only left the food on my plate that I thought would be a reasonable serving.

Well, after I finished eating what was on my plate...I was still hungry! It took almost 15 minutes before I started feeling full. And then I felt almost uncomfortably full.

It was a good reminder that feelings of fullness can take a long time to develop. Especially if you eat quickly, you can overshoot feeling normally "full" and get to "uncomfortably full and bloated" very easily.

Don't eat the extras at restaurants

Sometimes the actual restaurant meal is fine, and is a healthy choice. It only becomes too much when you eat the extras. The bread and butter set on the table when you first sit down, or the tortilla chips and salsa at Mexican restaurants. The appetizers, drinks and desserts—all of these together, on top of your main meal, can end up turning a reasonable meal into one that will make you gain weight.

I suggest, as a potential rule for you to consider, that you *always skip the extras* at a restaurant. Stick to the main meal, and skip whatever is on top of that—the drinks, bread, chips, appetizers, and dessert. Skipping the extras is an easy place to draw a line, and can make a good food rule.

Don't eat at fast food restaurants

Earlier, in the section on restaurants, one of the potential guidelines I gave was *Fast food can be okay*. And fast food *can* be okay—for some people. If you're able to occasionally stop at McDonald's and buy a regular cheeseburger and a cup of coffee—or whatever reasonable meal that you know is okay for you—that's perfectly fine.

But what if you eat many, many meals at fast food restaurants? What if you usually get the full-meal deal, and then "supersize" it, and get all kinds of extras?

In that case—maybe you need to avoid fast food restaurants entirely. Maybe you need to stay away from them, because they trigger eating behavior that you want to avoid.

In my research for this book, I reviewed some memoirs written by people who were extremely obese, and were trying to lose weight. And one thing that struck me was how many meals the authors ate at fast food restaurants. The combination of cheap food, speed and convenience (you can even stay in your car!) and delicious taste was hard to resist.

There are other food options that are similar to fast food restaurants in terms of bringing you delicious food, conveniently and cheaply. These are options like pizza delivery, or apps like Uber Eats and GrubHub that deliver restaurant food to you. They aren't as cheap, but they're still delicious and even more convenient. You need to consider carefully whether you should avoid them completely.

Drink only no-calorie drinks

Consider having a blanket rule, to avoid *all* drinks with calories.

This is a big, brute-force food rule. You'll want to tweak it to make it work for you. You may need lots of exceptions and adjustments. And you may need to work up to it gradually.

But it can be very powerful. And you can avoid lots of calories—calories that would give you zero nutrition, calories that would make it more difficult to lose weight and maintain your weight.

There's a whole section on drinks in the chapter, "Hazards you need to avoid". In that section, I give specifics on the types of drinks that you should be careful of, why they're dangerous, and how you could avoid them.

The principles when figuring out the specifics of your food rule for drinks are the same as for other food rules. Make it easy to avoid the things you should be avoiding. That means—don't buy sodas and other high-calorie drinks, don't have them in your home. Sports drinks, juices, and "healthy" smoothies are the same—they're promoted as healthier, but they're just as full of empty calories as soda. Avoid them.

You still want to be able to socialize, to visit a coffee shop with a friend. So, if you're avoiding the high-calorie lattes, mochas, and macchiatos, what do you drink instead?

The answer is simple. Regular coffee, black tea or herbal tea is just fine. People have been drinking these for hundreds of years.

Coffee, unsweetened, may seem too bitter. You may want to switch to a milder coffee blend. Or—sweeten your coffee or tea with a packet or two of sugar. It's fine to add *some* sugar in your coffee or tea, if you're transitioning away from heavily sweetened coffee drinks. It would be a very big jump to go from a super-sweet drink like a Caramel Brulée Latte to plain, unsweetened black coffee.

But try to transition to lightly sweetened coffee. It will be just as satisfying in a few months. And—as a bonus for making that switch—you'll start discovering sweetness in many other foods that didn't taste sweet before.

When it comes to juice, you may not want to avoid it completely. That's totally fine. If you must have juice, consider making your own. You can easily make orange and grapefruit juice with an inexpensive manual citrus juicer. It's very straightforward—but of course, it's more effort than just opening a container of juice. Squeezing one orange will leave you with about a third of a cup of juice. The effort involved—the fact that you have to put a little labor into it—makes you drink less. Which, in the case of juice, is a good thing. You may decide to just eat the orange instead of juicing it, which would be healthier anyway.

***

Here's my own, personal food rules for drinks. I drink coffee, tea, milk, water, juice that I make myself, and occasionally some wine. I avoid other drinks like soda, artificially sweetened drinks, purchased smoothies, etc. I sometimes make my own smoothies (usually with milk and some frozen fruit).

I will occasionally add some cream or sugar to my coffee, but I generally drink it black. And that wasn't an instant transition—I added one or two teaspoons of sugar to my coffee for months before I started drinking it black. I don't enjoy alcohol very much, so I don't really need any limits there. I don't drink skim milk or low-fat milk. I did, back when low-fat was very popular, but now I stick to regular whole milk.

I don't feel deprived by these rules. And there's no drink that I want, but can't have. My rules developed over time. You can also, over time, figure out your own personal rules related to drinks.

Alcohol, in particular, is a tricky thing for many people. You may want to have a strict daily limit, or a strict weekly limit. Alcohol has a *lot* of calories, and is often the gateway to overindulging on food. These are all things to keep in mind when you're trying to figure out your rules.

Here's a few more drink-related food rule ideas, from the chapter *Hazards You Need to Avoid.*

- Avoid soda
- Avoid fruit drinks and fruit juices
- Avoid "healthy" drinks, like smoothies and sweetened teas
- Avoid artificial sweeteners
- Avoid sweetened coffee drinks
- Limit alcohol

Junk foods only on weekends

One rule to consider is to only eat junk food (highly processed foods, salty treats, sweets, etc.) on weekends.

If you decide to follow this rule, you'd avoid foods like pastries, cookies, sugary cereal, chips and crackers, ice cream—but only on weekdays. On weekends, you'd be free to indulge in them.

This may be a reasonable rule for you to consider. There's a diet called the "No S Diet" (more info at NoSdiet.com) that incorporates this rule, as well as a few others, into a very concise set of rules:

- No Snacks
- No Sweets
- No Seconds
- Except (sometimes) on days that start with "S"

So, on Saturday and Sunday, you can break the "no snacks, no sweets, and no seconds" rule.

These rules, and variations on them, could be helpful to some people. You may be one of them.

I appreciate the conciseness of the No S Diet system, but I think most people would need some adjustments and tweaks. For instance, I don't like the idea of two out of seven days of the week being an "anything goes" day. A special day that comes along less often (birthdays, Christmas, etc.) would probably work better.

You could adjust this rule, too. Perhaps it could be something like "One serving of junk food is okay every weekend". That might work better a rule that says "Any junk food can be consumed on weekends".

Some things to consider, if you want to create a rule like this, are—would you keep junk food in the house, all through the week? That would be tempting, on the days you're not supposed to eat them.

No eating between meals

Here's another rule that works for many people, and may work for you. Basically, you eat only three meals a day, breakfast, lunch, and dinner. You eat nothing between meals.

So, no snacking. Since most people snack on unhealthy foods, you'll be reducing your calories if you follow this rule. And not eating between meals will mean that you're hungry before your next meal. You'll get used to the feeling of hunger—that it's not an emergency, and that it's something you can deal with.

This has the potential for being a good rule. It turns out that snacking—eating between meals—is actually a very new eating habit, and very closely linked to weight gain. According to some government studies, *most* of the extra calories added to the American diet in the past fifty or so years are from snacks.

The whole concept of regularly eating snacks is new. And the number of products specifically designed for snacking has exploded recently. Potato chips were invented in the 1800s. But only in the 1920s did they start to be sold in individual bags, that could be stored, and eaten conveniently as a snack. Before then, they were scooped from a barrel into a paper bag, and were often stale or crushed. And it was only in the late 1950s that flavoring was first added to potato chips, starting with Lay's Barbecue-flavored potato chips.

Now we have dozens, if not hundreds, of potato chips flavors available. With just a little bit of searching online, I was able to find a brand (Kettle) that has at least 16 flavors, among them Backyard BBQ, Jalapeno, Korean BBQ, New York Cheddar, Pepperoncini, Salt & Pepper, and Sea Salt & Vinegar.

These are the foods that most people snack on—hyperpalatable foods that are very hard to stop eating. Foods that have no nutritional value, other than excess calories we don't need.

These days, as a reaction to the very unhealthy snack foods that most people are eating, there's a trend towards more "healthy" snack foods. But these are mostly in the form of bars of some sort (energy bars, protein bars, etc.), or foods that are supposed to be a healthy substitute for potato chips (i.e. sweet potato chips). They're still just as unhealthy, and just as easy to overeat. And they're packed with as many calories as the snack food that they're substituting for.

✳✳✳

I still snack between meals, myself. But since I (mostly) avoid highly processed foods, all my snacks are either something I consider healthy (fruits or nuts), or a "junk food" that I've made myself (homemade cookies, popcorn, etc.).

None of these are foods that I would overeat. I wouldn't overeat fruit because it's bulky, and I just never want to eat more than one piece of fruit at a time. Nuts are a little trickier, especially flavored nuts, so I generally stick with plain almonds or peanuts, since I don't go overboard with them.

And since I actually made the homemade cookies and popcorn myself, it puts the brakes on how much I eat, because it takes some effort. Also, the rest of my family wants to eat them as well. Those two things naturally limit how much I eat, without needing to use my willpower.

This works for me, because I've made the decision to avoid highly processed foods. So, I eat almost none of the commonly eaten snack foods.

What about you? Would not eating between meals—no snacking—be a good rule, for you?

If you're eating highly processed foods, then yes, potentially this could be a very good rule for you. You're much more likely to eat the worst of the snack foods (for instance, a candy bar, or a bag of chips) as a snack, instead of at a meal. So, if you don't snack, you may be reducing the number of calories you eat.

As usual, only your daily weigh-in will tell you for sure, over time, if this is a good rule for you.

A potential exception may be fresh fruits. An apple or banana between meals could be a healthy addition to your diet, and they won't tempt you to overeat.

Nuts are a lot trickier, because they're very high in calories. But it's still worthwhile to figure out if there's a type of nut that's satisfying as a snack, but doesn't tempt you to overeat. For me, that's plain nuts (usually almonds or peanuts), instead of spiced, roasted nuts.

***

For me, the whole idea of having my own personal food rules started with french fries. I love french fries, but I also knew that I have a tendency to eat too many of them. And since they're so high in calories, that was a problem. I was sometimes able to limit how many I ate, but at the cost of stress and anxiety. And my weight was slowly creeping up. Of course, it wasn't *all* because of too many french fries, but they added to the problem.

Then I remembered the chapter about abstinence, in Gretchen Rubin's book *Better Than Before*. Her sister had resolved that she would be "Free from french fries", and I decided to give that a try. My idea was that it would be a temporary rule, and if I didn't like it, I would indulge in french fries again.

And that's how I discovered the power of having my own personal food rule. Once I had a rule that I had committed to follow, it was *so easy* to avoid french fries. There was no anxiety, there was no decision-making. It was completely different from trying to eat only *some* french fries. Avoiding them completely made life much easier, and knew I could keep it up forever.

After that, I decided to expand my rules, and avoid highly processed foods (with some exceptions). That worked well. Keeping my weight at the level I wanted much easier.

✳✳✳

I've given you a lot of potential food rules to consider. How do you pick which ones would work best for you? This is a very personal decision, and it all depends on your lifestyle and preferences.

I suggest that you move slowly. Start with weighing yourself every day for a few weeks, and see how that looks. Your daily weigh-in may give you some ideas about what your first food rules should be

Your food rules do not need to have you completely avoid a particular food. My exception is always "It's okay if I make it myself". I like that because it makes the food I want to limit (say, french fries), less convenient—but if I really wanted to, I could make it, without "breaking my rule".

And changing a rule is completely fine. Not in the moment of temptation, not when you're actually faced with the food that you have a rule about. But say you have a rule *Eat a maximum of one restaurant meal a* week. You've decided that rule is too restrictive, and you have to turn down too many invitations from friends if you follow it. So—change it. It's your personal food rule, and you're allowed to change it.

Your personal food rules will evolve over time. I started with *Don't eat french fries* and then within a few months added *Don't eat highly processed foods*. This works for me. Your food rules will be different.

Food Rules Summary

Below is a summary of the food rules from earlier in the chapter. Use them as a jumping-off point for your own food rules. Put a dot next to those that you're interested in, and a star next to those that you will try out.

Consider taping a list of the food rules you've decided on next to your weight chart.

_____ Don't eat french fries.

_____ Don't eat any fried foods.

_____ Don't eat any salty, highly processed snacks (fried, or otherwise).

_____ No sweets unless I made them myself.

_____ Don't buy any foods with added sugar.

_____ I make my own junk food.

_____ Eat one type of chocolate.

_____ Don't eat free food.

_____ Don't eat highly processed foods.

_____ Never eat food from a vending machine.

_____ Don't eat your trigger foods.

_____ Don't eat after dinner.

_____ Eat a maximum of one restaurant meal a week.

_____ Before starting your meal at a restaurant, put some of it in a take-out container.

_____ Don't eat the extras at restaurants.

_____ Don't eat at fast food restaurants.

_____ Drink only no-calorie drinks.

_____ Junk foods only on weekends.

_____ No eating between meals.

_____ My personal food rule #1:

_____

_____ My personal food rule #2:

_____

_____ My personal food rule #3:

_____

FOOD RULES: QUESTIONS AND ANSWERS

Some common questions like "What if I break my own food rules", and "How long should I follow my food rules?"

The food environment we have in today's world is really good at tempting and stimulating people to eat, far more than what their body needs.

But "the food environment we have in today's world" does not need to be *your* food environment. You create your own, personal food rules—and this is how you create your own, personal food environment.

By creating food rules like *I only eat junk food that I make myself,* you erase a whole category of foods that are causing obesity. When you follow this food rule, then purchased junk foods don't exist for you. You've changed your own, personal food environment, so it gives you a better chance of losing weight, and staying at a healthier weight.

It takes effort, though. This is not how most people live. Here's some of the questions that can commonly come up about food rules.

How do I pick my food rules?

Hopefully the last chapter, with a long list of food rules to consider, gives you some ideas. What are some strategies you can use, to decide on the best food rules for you to start with? Here's a few thoughts.

One strategy is to **target the worst food habit you have**. If it's buying food from fast food restaurants regularly, your first food rule may be *Never eat at fast food restaurants*. This would mean a big change, but maybe you're up for a big change.

Maybe a strategy like that is too big a step. Perhaps you'd rather **target an easy win**. Say you go to coffee shops every day, and buy fancy sweetened drinks like Caramel Cloud Macchiato or Pumpkin Spice Latte. Maybe your rule would be *Never buy anything but plain coffee or tea at a coffee shop*. And you allow yourself to still add sugar or cream to the drink. Successfully following this rule gives you the confidence to add more rules.

When you're deciding on food rules, remember that at the beginning, you're experimenting. You want to figure out—is this a rule I could follow for a lifetime? That means it can't be too difficult, and it can't make you unhappy. It shouldn't prevent you from having a social life.

And remember also—the scale is the ultimate guide. If you're following your food rules but not losing any weight, then you need to change something.

What if I break my food rules?

Let's say you've thought carefully about your food rules, and now to create ones that work for you. You've considered your worst food habits and set up some rules that will counteract them, and reduce your calories. You're not testing out rules anymore, you're committed to them.

But then, in a moment of weakness or social pressure, you break one of your rules. What's the best way to deal with this?

The first thing to do is remember—this is not something that calls for any kind of "punishment". Doing a long session on the treadmill, if you think of it as "punishment", is not going to be useful. It won't help stick with your food rule.

You may be feeling guilty. I wrote earlier that guilt, blame, and shame can get in the way of the work that you need to do, in order to manage your weight. So, let any feelings of guilt, blame, or shame be short-term, temporary feelings. They can motivate you to find a strategy for sticking with your food rule. And then—let go. Guilt, blame, and shame have no long-term use.

Here's a few steps you can take to figure out how you can solve your problem and stick with your food rule:

Weigh yourself tomorrow morning. Keep weighing yourself every day, and logging it. This is the foundation; this is how you keep yourself honest. Breaking your food rule is a mistake, not a catastrophe. But keep weighing yourself daily.

Analyze what went wrong with the rule, and consider changing it. Think like a detective. What was the situation in which you broke your rule? Were you trying to use willpower and/or moderation? Was there alcohol involved? Did you have an exception to your rule that was too broad?

For instance, say your rule is *No junk food except on weekends*. But maybe eating junk food on Saturday and Sunday keeps you trapped in a junk food addiction, which makes weekdays too hard. So, you may want to remove that exception.

Or maybe you need to change a rule by actually *making* an exception. Maybe your rule is *No junk food*. And that feels too hard, like you never get to enjoy any treats. In that case, maybe you want to change your rule to *No junk food, except what I make for myself.*

It's also possible that the rule is fine, and you don't need to make any changes. Perhaps you just need to recommit, 100%.

Think about making it impossible to break your food rule. Maybe your rule is *No food from vending machines*. But in a moment of weakness or stress, you bought some food from a vending machine.

What do you need to do, so that you don't rely on willpower? How could you make it, so that you literally could *not* buy food from the vending machine? Figure out what would work, and do that. Maybe you need to only bring larger bills, that can't be used in vending machines? Or maybe you need to leave all your cash at home?

226

Think of a slogan for yourself. This doesn't need to be anything fancy. But pick a few motivational phrases that you can inspire yourself with, when facing a difficult moment. For instance:

I'll feel better tomorrow if I stick to my rule

There is no choice—I have my rule

Tomorrow morning I'll be stepping on the scale

Also—remember the "Why I want to lose weight" list that you made earlier? Consider writing them on an index card, and keeping them with you. Or, put them on the home page of your phone—whatever works for you. Anything that reminds you of your long-term goals is a good thing. You want to be thinking of where you want to be in 6 months, instead of the immediate pleasure of food.

Write down your rules. If you haven't yet written down your rules, do that now. You can tape them up next to your weight chart, or put them in a notebook. Consider writing them by hand, instead of typing it and printing it out. Writing things out by hand makes your rule more real, and easier to remember. It solidifies them in your mind, and makes you more committed.

How long should I follow my food rules?

You know the answer to this one, but let's talk about it anyway. You need to follow your food rules...*forever*. They are your lifetime food rules. These are not rules someone else told you to follow—they're your own, personalized food rules. You can adjust them when you decide they need adjustment, but in general, they're lifetime rules.

Most people don't have food rules. They're doing what people have done for millennia, which is just eating whatever tempting foods are around. And this has been the right choice, for a very long time.

But now, the world has changed. Our food environment has changed. Today, eating whatever is tasty and available leads to being overweight or obese. And this is not just for a few, vulnerable people, with "low willpower"—this is for *most* people.

Your food rules help you build a wall between you and today's toxic food environment. When you take your food rules seriously, you actually *change* your food environment to one that's much healthier.

To give you an idea of how this works, let's say that, like many people, you're exposed to free food many times a day. For example, you often have free pastries at your workplace in the mornings, and then free food samples at the grocery store after work.

But if you have a rule for yourself, that says *I don't eat free food*—you've changed your food environment. Once your rule is solid, once you believe in your ability to follow it without stress, then you're golden. Those extra 500 calories of "free food" that you would have eaten without thinking—they disappear. And then you can lose weight, or keep the weight off.

Your food rules are like a wall, separating you from the current food environment. Every day that you follow your food rules, you add another brick to the wall. And that wall needs to stay there for a lifetime.

✱✱✱

Recently I made Easter baskets for my kids. This meant taking large bags of candy, and dividing the candies up into lots of little plastic Easter eggs that I then hid around the yard. So, I was actually touching the tempting candy dozens and dozens of times, filling up each egg.

That was challenging, because eating these candies would have broken a food rule. One of my food rules is *Don't eat highly processed foods,* and candies are a highly processed food. I make some exceptions, but these candies were not one of them. So, just eating whatever candies that I happen to run across is not okay.

These are some of the most tempting situations around. Having a tempting food *in your hand* and not eating it is challenging. What helped me resist was knowing these things:

- I can have candy, just not this particular candy.
- Following a food rule strictly makes it much easier, over the long run, to keep weight off.

It's best to avoid tempting situations if you can. In general—especially at the beginning—I recommend avoiding temptation, or making it impossible to break your food rule.

But once you've been in a tempting situation like this, and *still* followed your food rule, the rule becomes much stronger. Your food rule gives you a wall, that separates you from the toxic food environment. And when you follow the rule even in a challenging situation, you make that wall stronger. The next time you're faced with temptation, you have a history of following your rule, and it gets much easier.

What if I feel like I'm missing out?

Fear of missing out, or FOMO, is a subject that we've heard a lot about recently. These days, in the era of social media, we're constantly aware of what other people are doing and eating.

So, when you set up food rules that prevent you from eating what everyone else is eating, you may feel like you're missing out. Say, for example, you have the rule: *No junk food unless I make it myself.* But today, at your office, somebody is having a birthday and there's a huge assortment of tempting cupcakes. The cupcakes are piled high with colorful frosting and various toppings. It looks like everyone is indulging, except you.

What can you do, to help you get through those feelings? Here's a few things to remember.

These feelings are temporary. As soon as you're away from the immediate temptation, when the food is right in front of you, you probably won't even think about it. Plenty of people will have regrets if they *do* indulge in the cupcakes. But if you skip the cupcake, you will not have any regrets. And over time, once you've faced these types of temptations many times, and stuck to your rule, it'll get much easier.

You can make it yourself. Whatever you're tempted by—it's possible to make it at home. It may require some work in the kitchen, but it can be done.

Understand the seriousness of the obesity problem. It's important to really understand at a gut level, how different the food environment is from earlier times. Highly tempting foods like these cupcakes are much more available than they were earlier. And the situation above, with the cupcakes, is exactly the type of situation that's contributing to our massive obesity problem. Consider reviewing the chapter *The History of Obesity* if you need to remind yourself how these foods can lead directly to obesity.

These are *your* food rules. You designed them; you made the decision to put them in your life. And you can change them, if need be (though not in a moment of temptation, of course). You don't need to miss out on anything that will truly make your life better—and you can set up your food rules so that you don't. But eating a random cupcake will not make your life better. If you really desire a sweet treat, take some time and make it yourself.

These foods are designed to be addictive. New, highly processed and delicious foods are constantly being developed. Tens of thousands of new food products come onto the market every year, according to the United States Department of Agriculture. Most of them are flops, but the ones that succeed are those that are the most addictive and appealing. These foods are designed to be as delicious and convenient as possible. Thousands of hours of laboratory research and testing are put into them.

Do you want to be the lab rat in this experiment? No, you don't. Make a decision to draw the line, and stick to your food rule.

Do I have to make big changes right away, or can I break it into small steps?

No, you don't have to make big changes right away. It's much better to break it down into smaller steps. An exception to this is if you have an addiction to something like fast food, or convenience store food. If this is your situation, you may need to completely stop going to fast food stores, or convenience stores.

The quote below was done up in cross-stitch, and framed on my piano teacher's living room wall when I was about 10. I've remembered it ever since.

Inch by inch, life's a cinch. Yard by yard, life is hard.
— John Bytheway

What it means to me is—don't demand perfection. The way to lose weight, and manage your weight over time, is to take small steps that improve your habits. Figure out which small steps work best. Then keep on taking them—and figure out your next step.

As a nation, the United States became obese slowly. Yes, you could say, "The obesity rate increased dramatically". But in the lives of actual people, these people gained weight slowly, over years and years. Gradually, over time, we ate at restaurants more. We cooked less. We started snacking more, and buying more and more highly processed, addictive convenience foods. And over time, these habit changes led to obesity.

Reversing these habits is not automatic. You need to take it step-by-step, because massive lifestyle changes don't work. Earlier in this book, I wrote about the reality TV show *The Biggest Loser*. Participants lived away from their homes. Their food and exercise habits were *completely* overhauled in a new environment, and they lost massive amounts of weight. But these new habits fell apart when went home, and they usually regained most of their weight.

Here's the type of small steps that can work. These small steps add up—over time—to large lifestyle changes.

- **You become convinced that you need to weigh yourself daily**. You buy a scale, tape some graph paper to the wall, and start weighing yourself every day. Your daily weigh-in takes just a few seconds.
- **You start noticing food temptations around you**. In the back of your mind, you're thinking about changes you could make. In your office, you become aware that there's always tempting sweets around. You consider making some of it out-of-bounds. You keep weighing yourself daily.
- You make a list of the specific reasons you want to lose weight. This list stays in your pocket, and you look at it occasionally.
- **You decide to try out some personal food rules**. Your first ones are *No sweets unless I made them myself* and *I don't eat fried foods,* for one month.
- **Breakfast has not been a good meal for you.** You want to improve it, so you decide to switch out your daily coffee shop/croissant habit, and have something healthier. You make a bowl of oatmeal in the microwave every day for a week, with some raisins and a little peanut butter. It's not bad.
- **You realize that over a month, you've lost 3 pounds**. It must be the food rules you set up (*No sweets unless I made them myself* and *I don't eat fried foods*) and the healthier breakfast. Also, you're probably cutting back on

233

overeating without thinking about it—maybe because you don't want to see jumps in your weight the next morning.

- **As a next step, you've been considering skipping lattes and other fancy coffee drinks**. Instead of those drinks, you'll just get black coffee with a packet of sugar when you go to the coffee shop. Your new food rule is *No fancy coffee drinks,* for a month, and see how it goes.

This is how food habit changes—the ones that stick—happen. The decision that you *will* lose weight may come quickly. But the actual habit changes may be slower. Figuring out how to drop your worst food habits, and how to replace them with healthier habits is a learning process. It takes time, and it's personal.

Here's the food rules that were put into place in the above scenario.

- No sweets unless I made them myself
- I don't eat fried foods
- No fancy coffee drinks

These rules develop over time. They're a way to guide and direct your food habits. Rules prevent you from needing to make a decision, every time you're faced with a food you want to avoid. You've pre-made the decision—you have a rule.

Weighing yourself daily is a critical step in the learning process. Without it, you don't know for sure which habits and food rules are helpful, and which aren't.

If I had rushed the diet, as I had done during previous attempts to lose weight, I never would have developed the necessary habits that enable me to go on eating less in a

Here's how the small steps might work if you've decided that you want to improve your breakfast routine. Your current habit is to have a bowl of sugary cereal at home.

- You switch to a less sugary cereal, like plain Cheerios. You add lots of sugar because without sugar, it tastes strange to you.
- You decide you can eat the Cheerios with just one level teaspoon of sugar, and add a sliced banana.
- You find an easy oatmeal recipe, and start making yourself homemade oatmeal. You add some fresh or frozen fruit, and a few nuts or some butter.

In this scenario, maybe you now decide that you'll have a food rule—*I don't eat packaged breakfast cereal*. This could be a baby step in the direction of *I don't eat highly processed foods*. Or not—only you can decide.

Say you want to improve how you eat when you're at work, in your office. Your current habit is to eat whatever free food is available at work, and also to get one or more snacks from the vending machines at work. This is how a gradual, sustainable habit can look:

- You decide to try out *I don't eat free food at work* and *I don't buy food from the vending machine for a month*. And you make it impossible to buy anything from the

235

vending machine by removing the dollar bills from your wallet, and keeping only an emergency $50 bill.

- You bring a packaged granola bar from home every day, and eat that instead of candy bars or chips from the vending machine. The granola bar is not the healthiest food around, but it's better than chips or a candy bar.
- You decide you need to eat more fruits and vegetables, so you stop bringing granola bars to work, and bring a piece of fruit to work every day. You also have some almonds in your drawer at work, to round out your snack.

These types of small changes are the ones that you'll be able to sustain over time. Paired with your lifelong habit of weighing yourself daily, you learn what works and what doesn't. And you'll adjust your food rules and habits, to make it work.

I am doing much better just making small adjustments— adapting over time, and adding new ones, than I ever did with going full-blown food reset, whole foods only, working out 4 times a week, in a huge "overhaul".
—From the online forum Reddit LoseIt

✳✳✳

How is this "small steps" approach different from moderation? I don't believe in moderation as a good strategy for weight management. Most people think of moderation in terms of never completely denying yourself anything. For instance, "I'll always have some potato chips around, but I'll just eat a few every day, instead of finishing the whole bag at once."

That has never worked for me, and it doesn't work for many people, perhaps most of them. These are all moderation techniques that are *not* effective:

- Using willpower to avoid junk foods
- "Listening to your body" to figure out when you should stop eating junk food
- Only eating a "reasonable portion" of a highly addictive food

What *does* work is drawing bright lines between the habit you want, and the one you don't want. For instance, rules like *I only eat salty snacks if I make them myself.*

A food rule that does involve using moderation could be something like *I have one serving of chips, once a week, and keep nothing at home.* So, you're still eating the really tempting, highly processed food, but controlling the amount, and not keeping it at home. That could work, perhaps. Only you can know for sure, and you can only know this over time. But in general, I would suggest caution with food rules that involve moderation. These are the rules that open the door to highly tempting foods just a little bit, and then shut it again. It may be better, in the long run, to choose a rule like *I only eat chips that I make myself.*

Small steps are different from moderation. A small step is not, "I'll keep the Oreo cookies around, I just won't eat as many". It should not involve willpower. And it does not ask you to always face temptation and decide, when facing that temptation, if you should indulge yourself.

Say you've decided to make your breakfast healthier, and you're switching from a high-sugar cereal to one with no added sugar. Would you just put the healthier cereal right next to the sugary cereal, look at both of them every morning, and use your willpower to choose the healthier one? No, you *throw away the sugary cereal*. You've already decided, and you don't want to be faced with making a new choice every morning.

Here's a list of small steps you could take, if you're trying to limit your calories from coffee drinks:

- Before you make any changes, you're regularly drinking large sizes of sugary, creamy hot coffee drinks (such as Pumpkin Spice Latte, Caramel Frappuccino, etc.).
- You switch to plain coffee or tea. Add as much sugar and cream as you like, but add it yourself.
- Coffee or tea. Add 1 package (1 level teaspoon) of sugar.
- Coffee or tea, with no added sugar. Tea is easy to drink this way, but black coffee may taste a little bitter, depending on whether it's a dark or light roast.

The last step—no added sugar—isn't necessary, but I would suggest that you stick to 1 teaspoon of sugar or less.

You can use this "small-steps" approach to adjust all your food habits, starting with the worst ones. The plan doesn't need to be completely thought out in advance. You just need to be willing to regularly take a small step in the right direction. And these are not meant to be steps that are hard or stressful, or make you feel deprived.

Remember—your goal here is to gradually make the small steps that *you could be happy with, for a lifetime*.

Summary

- When choosing your personal food rules, think long-term. You're testing the rule out, to see if you could follow it forever, and if it helps you lose weight.
- If you break a personal food rule:
  - Keep on weighing yourself daily.
  - Analyze the rule, and consider changing it. Is it too strict? Too easy to break?
  - Think about making it impossible to break your rule.
  - Write down your rules.
  - Think of a motivational slogan for yourself.
- Your personal food rules are for a lifetime. You can make exceptions, and you can change your rules. But in general, for lifetime weight management, you need lifetime food rules.
- If you're worried that you're missing out, here are some thoughts to consider:
  - These feelings will go away.
  - You can make it yourself.
  - Understand how dangerous the obesity problem is.
  - These are *your* food rules.
  - These foods are designed to be addictive.
- You do not need to make big changes all at once. Don't rush it, and feel free to take the food rules one step at a time.

FOOD GUIDELINES

---

*Sane principles and guidelines to
help you handle our insane food
environment*

What are food guidelines? And how are they different from food rules?

In the previous chapters, I went into detail on one of the most important strategies for managing your weight—your personal food rules. The food rules are restrictions that you set up, for yourself. By restricting your options, you make it easier to avoid unhealthy food choices, without stress.

A food rule is something like *I don't keep packaged sweet snacks at home*. This is a personal food rule that you've decided on, because you have a hard time not eating sweets when they're convenient. You can make exceptions if you want, but in general, it's straightforward. It's easy to know if you're following it, or not.

Food guidelines, on the other hand, are universal. They're basic principles and advice that apply to everyone, and can help you figure out how you can eat differently. They help you when you're figuring out your personal food rules, but they're not rules. For instance, the guideline *One slice of bread instead of two* is a reminder that the amount of food you eat matters. And the guideline *Make the right choice convenient, make the wrong choice inconvenient* could convince you to create a rule like *I will not keep packaged snack food in my desk at work.*

If your rules aren't working, change them

I've mentioned this in passing before, but it's worthwhile being 100% clear about it. If you're working on losing weight and you're not losing even a small amount of weight in a week, then you want to think about changing your rules.

If you're working at maintaining your weight, but you're very slowly gaining weight—again, something needs to change.

Figuring out the right rule change takes thought. The new or updated rule needs to:

- Lower the number of calories you're taking in
- Work over the long term
- Not be too hard to follow

And the right rule change is different for everyone. For some people, constantly having tempting snacks and treats at the workplace is a killer. Maybe your rule should be *I don't eat free food at work.*

Or if snacking after dinner is your problem, think about how you could limit or completely avoid that type of eating. Maybe a rule like *I only eat fruit after dinner* would help.

Variety is your enemy. Routine is your friend.

This guideline may seem counterintuitive—how could variety be the enemy? You may be thinking, "Variety is famous for being 'the spice of life'—what's wrong with it?"

And I'm sure you've seen these types of messages over and over again:

Choose a variety of foods from each food group to build healthy eating styles.

Eating a variety of foods promotes good health and can help reduce the risk of disease.

The *intention* behind this type of advice is that people should not just eat plain oatmeal for breakfast. They should eat oatmeal, but with raisins, sliced bananas, and milk. Or, instead of a piece of toast for lunch, they would eat toast with some peanut butter, and fresh fruit on the side. In other words, a healthier, balanced meal.

That's the intention. What's been happening, though? People are eating a lot of variety, but it's a variety of highly processed junk foods. So, instead of just ordering the Ultimate Pepperoni Pizza from Dominos, they order the Ultimate Pepperoni Pizza along with a side of Cinnamon Bread Twists. The variety consists of two highly processed, highly addictive foods instead of one.

Earlier in this book, in the section about variety in food, I mentioned sensory-specific satiety. This is also known as the buffet effect. It's easy to visualize this effect in your own life, because it takes place all the time. Say you're eating a food you love—for

243

instance, chocolate pudding. You're hungry, and you have a lot of pudding available, so you eat a large amount. But eventually, you get tired of it. You're done with it, and wouldn't want to eat another bite.

However, if now you had some potato chips available—could you eat more? Sure. It's a completely different taste, and a different feel in your mouth. You could eat a lot more.

And, of course, this effect is magnified, depending on how many different foods are offered. That's how the name the "buffet effect" came about. At a buffet, you have a huge variety of tasty foods. And people often overeat, by a massive amount. They will often eat double, triple, or even more than what they would eat at a normal meal.

How can knowing about the buffet effect help you manage your weight? The title of this section says it all:

Variety is your enemy. Routine is your friend.

In other words—you need to take the danger of variety seriously. In the food environment that we have today, most of the food variety is the type you should avoid completely. For instance, below are just a few of the currently available Cheetos snack varieties:

CHEETOS® Crunchy Cheese
CHEETOS® Puffs Cheese Flavored Snacks
CHEETOS® Crunchy FLAMIN' HOT® Chipotle Ranch
CHEETOS® Paws Cheese Flavored Snacks

244

For me, many of these snacks sound delicious. I've always had a weakness for crunchy, cheesy snacks. I know for a fact that they would be tasty.

But I know a few other things, too. They are:

- These products are designed to be addictive. It's best not to start on them.
- I'm not missing out if I avoid them—I can make my own salty snacks.
- Most people who eat these foods gain weight.

✳✳✳

The Cheetos products listed above are just an example of the type of variety that surrounds us. And *all* of this variety needs to be avoided. Most of it is just part of the constant churning out of new products by food manufacturers and restaurants. They're trying to get us hooked on them, trying to get these new products to be part of our life.

The flip side of variety is routine. And that's what I'm recommending. I'm recommending that you develop some routine meals. These need to be meals that you find appealing, and convenient. You're fine with eating them multiple times a week. They should be reasonably healthy. And, importantly, it needs to be easy to eat whatever amount that's right for you.

This means that you may eat some of the same meals often. But what if that's not appealing to you? What if trying new restaurants and novel foods is a big part of your life? Routine can sound boring.

If this is the case for you, try directing that desire for novelty to a different path. For instance—cooking at home, and trying new recipes. Most people that have lost weight and are keeping it off eat at home much more often than average. They eat many fewer restaurant meals.

And these people often have default, go-to meals. These are meals for which you always have the ingredients at home, and can put together relatively quickly. And they substitute for unhealthy alternatives. For instance, you could have a healthy default breakfast of oatmeal with sliced bananas and some chopped walnuts. This could substitute for a sugary latte and croissant from the coffee shop. Or—on evenings when you're pressed for time, you scramble a few eggs, and have some toast, instead of a default dinner of take-out Chinese food.

✳✳✳

Human beings are driven to want variety in their food. This was useful, throughout human history. It helped us survive. Just as we have an instinct to eat high-calorie foods, we also have an instinct to eat a variety of foods. But many years ago, this would have meant something different from what it does today. This drive for variety would have encouraged us to eat a bowl of lentil soup, in addition to some bread. Or, it would have pushed us to search for and eat fruits whenever they were available, because they weren't an everyday food. So, our instinct for variety gave us better nutrition.

The variety that we're offered today is different, though. Now, our natural drive to eat a variety of food has been hijacked. The variety of foods that we're offered today offer nothing but *taste* variety. They do not offer variety in nutrition.

Having routines can be just as helpful for weight management as having food rules. Food rules eliminate choices, and so do routines. If your standard breakfast routine is a bowl of oatmeal with some milk and fruit, then you eliminate the need to make choices. You've already made your decision.

Say you have, for instance, ten routine, healthy meals that you like, and you mostly alternate between them. If you do this, you're going to be eating a relatively healthy diet. You'll be on the path to managing your weight—either losing weight if you need to, or maintaining your weight.

One slice of bread instead of two

Years ago, whenever I made myself scrambled eggs, I'd make two eggs, and toast two slices of bread with them. That was one of my routine meals. This was in my twenties, when I had jobs that kept me more physically active. So, I probably needed the extra calories.

I kept up this routine when I was in my thirties. Two eggs, two slices of bread. But it became obvious that it was *too much*. It wasn't extreme, it was just a few too many calories. Two slices were more than I needed for a routine meal. So, I switched to one slice, and two eggs. And that's right for me, now.

This type of situation happens a lot. We eat the "normal" amount, or whatever is put in front of us. We don't evaluate—is this the right amount for me?

Over the months and years, if most meals are like this—each one with a few too many calories—you gain weight. This is especially easy to do if you're not weighing yourself daily.

So, figure out if your regular meals are a reasonable size, for you. Maybe you normally have a sandwich for lunch every day, with two slices of bread. You may need to switch to a half sandwich, with one slice of bread, and a side of fruit or soup.

✳✳✳

Obviously, the bread in "One slice of bread instead of two" is just a stand-in for whatever type of food might be too much. Say you love wine, and have two glasses of wine every evening. Maybe you need to switch to one glass of wine.

I have a bowl of oatmeal for breakfast most mornings. It's not a very low-calorie meal, since as well as fruits, I also put peanut butter and various nuts in it. So, even though it's very healthy, I don't want to eat too much.

It can be a hassle to stir up the oatmeal, and mix in all the fruits and nuts in my regular-sized bowl. So, I switched to a larger bowl—kind of a pasta bowl. And that made it much easier to stir.

But something else happened as well. I switched to a larger bowl—and somehow, automatically, I filled it up more. I ended up with about a third more food in my bowl. I love my oatmeal, but that was just too much. So, I switched back to the regular size bowl. It's still a pain to stir things up in a smaller bowl, but using it automatically controls how much I eat. And since this is such a routine breakfast for me, I need to eat a reasonable quantity.

The quantity of what you're eating matters—a lot. Especially for the routine meals that you eat all the time, make sure the amount is reasonable for you. Switching the size of your plate or bowl or glass may be helpful.

Hunger before meals is normal

The abundance of food that we have now is a new situation. And hunger, which has existed for millions of years, cannot deal with it. Hunger tells us to eat. Why shouldn't it? Through all of human history, eating whenever food was available was the right choice. The feeling of hunger that pushed us to eat was a trustworthy guide to survival.

Not anymore. Now, hunger is telling us to eat more, when eating more is the wrong choice for our health. It's pushing us to eat more even when that can lead to weight gain, and illnesses like diabetes. Today, hunger is not a reliable guide to how much you should eat. This is especially the case when you have a variety of appetizing foods in front of you.

Is there anything pushing us to stop eating—a feeling that's the opposite of hunger? There's the uncomfortable feeling of being bloated, but that only comes when you've eaten far, far more than you need. It doesn't prevent you from eating the extra 200 or so daily calories that lead to slow weight gain.

There was recently an ad for Snickers with the slogan, "You're Not You When You're Hungry". These types of ads encourage us to believe that hunger is an abnormal feeling, and it needs to be fixed immediately. They imply that if you're hungry, you're not yourself, and you should stop right away to eat a Snickers bar.

That's what advertisers would like you to believe, but it's not true. Hunger is a complex instinct, as well as an emotional state. It's much, much stronger when appetizing food is around.

Hunger is also normal, even though snack food manufacturers would like you to believe that it's not. If you're not regularly hungry, every day, before at least a few meals, then you're probably slowly gaining weight.

Many diet programs and books claim to help you "lose weight without hunger". But they're promising something they can't deliver. Hunger is a normal part of daily life. Every day, you should experience hunger. This is not extreme hunger, that you suffer from for hours and hours, but normal hunger—the type that you get before meals.

At the beginning of your weight loss, hunger may be difficult to deal with. This is especially true if your old habit was to eat something as soon as you felt any hunger. If you haven't experienced normal hunger in a while, you may have developed a fear of it.

Here's some ideas on dealing with hunger. Hunger is personal. You need to learn to deal with it on a personal level, and figure out which approach works best for you.

Review your "Why I want to lose weight" list. Earlier I suggested that you write a detailed, personal list of the reasons that you want to lose weight. Read and review this list. This can be a powerful antidote to hunger. It will help you wait for your next planned meal.

Distract yourself. Talking to someone on the phone, cleaning the kitchen, taking a walk, doing the laundry. Doing something physical, something active, can be a great distraction from hunger.

Make yourself some tea. Having something to drink gives you something to do with your hands, and distracts you. It's a myth that people mistake thirst for hunger, and therefore drinking something can relieve hunger. But still, having something to drink is a great distraction. It doesn't need to be tea, just something with no calories, or low-calorie.

Make it impossible to get a snack that you shouldn't be eating. If you're often tempted by things like candy bars in a vending machine—leave the cash at home, or in your car. The specifics of this will depend on your situation, but try to make it *impossible* to buy the foods you should avoid. You may not need to do this forever, but it will help in the first months, as you're learning how to manage hunger.

Have a not-very-tempting snack available. If you're having a very hard time dealing with hunger, consider having a snack available. I'm not talking about something highly processed, like a protein bar, chips, or something similar. I'm suggesting something basic, like a banana or a hard-boiled egg. It should be something lower in calories, that you don't find highly tempting, but that you'll eat if you're very hungry.

Remember—hunger is normal. If you're losing weight, you're going to be experiencing hunger. Even if you're maintaining weight, it's normal to be hungry before meals.

Cook at home. Eat at home.

Unfortunately, cooking and eating at home is becoming less and less popular. Although the number of cooking shows (Top Chef, Master Chef, The Great British Baking Show, etc.) has increased dramatically, the number of people regularly cooking at home is going down. Watching these shows may even be decreasing people's desire to cook, because the shows make cooking seem highly stressful and complex. They're entertaining to watch, sure, but they don't make cooking seem like a normal part of life.

Cooking *should* be a normal part of life, though. It doesn't need to be difficult and complicated. It's possible to use only simple ingredients that are easy to find in a regular grocery store. You can have a few standard recipes that you make often, for most meals.

Learning to cook a few recipes, and eating mostly at home can be crucial for managing your weight. It helps you in many ways. Food you make yourself, at home, keeps you away from highly processed foods. It keeps you out of restaurants. And since highly processed foods and restaurants are two of the biggest hazards of today's food environment, avoiding them is critical.

Another way that making your own food helps control your weight is this: when you make a delicious, tempting food less convenient, you're much less likely to eat it. And of course, making the food yourself, instead of buying it, is definitely less convenient. It takes more time and work to produce the same food. This puts the brakes on consumption.

So, cooking for yourself has two main benefits for managing your weight:

- You avoid highly processed foods, and restaurant foods
- When you do want sweet treats, or salty snacks, it takes more work to make it at home, so you do it less often

You don't need to cook at home all the time. You don't need to completely avoid highly processed foods (although that may be right for you). You just need to lean more towards cooking and eating at home, and mostly making your own foods. This is the way almost everybody lived, 50 to 100 years ago. If you made a conscious decision to eat this way again—and made some personal rules or guidelines around this way of eating—you would be well along the path towards a healthy weight.

Since sweets and salty snack foods are some of the most addictive and tempting high-calorie foods around, you may want to consider learning how to make them yourself. This way, you could realistically have a rule like *I don't buy snack food.* Knowing a few good recipes for snack foods means still being able to have them occasionally, without buying the packaged versions.

✳✳✳

When you're cooking at home, it's perfectly fine to use frozen and canned foods. I saw one diet book that told readers to stay away from any food that needed to be defrosted, or needed a can opener. But that's a silly rule that just makes life more difficult, without helping you manage your weight.

For instance, I made homemade chili recently, using canned beans, and frozen ground beef. It went together very quickly, and I made a double batch, so I could freeze leftovers for another meal.

The alternative to using canned beans and frozen ground beef would have been to buy fresh ground beef (and use it up quickly, because otherwise it would spoil), and cook my own beans from scratch. It would have made the whole process take much longer, without making the meal healthier at all.

So yes—stay away from highly processed frozen foods like frozen waffles, or frozen chicken pot pie. Avoid canned ravioli and similar canned foods. But it's completely fine to use single-ingredient frozen foods, such as vegetables, fruits, meats, or seafoods. And many canned foods, like canned beans for my chili, are completely fine.

Fresh foods, if you're not used to them, can be tricky to use up before they go bad. Some fresh foods like carrots, cabbage, and potatoes will last for a very long time. But others (lettuce, tomatoes, berries) go bad much more quickly than others.

Start with just a few basic recipes, and give yourself time. It will take time and thought to make cooking at home a default choice, and a convenient one. But it will repay you over and over, throughout your lifetime.

Balance your plate

One of the ways of lowering the number of calories you eat is to eat less of a particular food. And the other is to eat the same amount—the same volume—but make that amount *lower in calorie density*.

What does that mean? The calorie density of a particular food is the number of calories per gram of that food. Take, for example, fruit. From lowest calorie density to highest calorie density in fruit, you'd go from a strawberry (low calorie density, .3 calories per gram) to avocado (high calorie density, 1.6 calories per gram). For dairy foods, you'd go from non-fat milk (.3 calories per gram) to parmesan cheese (4 calories per gram)

Calorie density is a useful concept, and it's good information to have. There's been a number of books written about it, such as *Volumetrics: Feel Full on Few Calories* by Barbara J. Rolls.

But the assumption is often made that *everything* you eat needs to be low in calorie density. So, the "good" foods are the ones low in calorie density, like non-fat milk. And the "bad" foods are the ones high in calorie density, like parmesan cheese.

This basically means you can only eat low-fat food. And only eating low-fat food is not sustainable. Most people can't keep that up for a lifetime.

The useful part of the calorie density concept is *not* that everything needs to be low in calorie density (i.e. low-fat). The thing to remember is that you should try to have a *balanced plate*. That means that for most meals, it's completely fine to have something that's higher in calorie density. Just balance it with something that's lower in calorie density.

For instance, say you're having an egg salad sandwich for lunch.

- It's fine to make it with full-fat mayonnaise instead of non-fat mayonnaise.
- You don't have to use just the low-fat egg whites—go ahead and use the whole egg. Much of the nutrition is in the yolk, anyway.
- You don't have to put extreme amounts of vegetables in the egg salad, so that there are more vegetables than eggs.

So, it's fine to make a standard recipe for an egg salad sandwich, not a low-fat version. You may potentially want to have a half sandwich instead of a whole, depending on your calorie needs.

But in any case, you should *balance your plate.* This means put some lower calorie items, usually fruits and vegetables, on your plate as well.

So, have some sliced apples or cucumbers on the side. Or a bowl of soup, or a small salad. Choose whatever works best for you, but balance your plate with some lower calorie foods.

You should put these additions *on your plate* before you start eating. Don't just assume you'll eat them later on, once you've finished the main part of your meal. You may not. And don't take seconds of the main part of the meal (in this case, the sandwich) until you've finished your sides.

Here's a few ways that balancing your plate will help you.

You reduce your calories

The main point of balancing your plate is to easily and comfortably lower the number of calories you're taking in. You're still eating a full meal, on a full plate. Yet you won't be overeating. And you'll still be lowering the total number of calories you're eating, compared to eating a full plate of higher calorie foods.

It's a habit you can keep up

Unlike switching completely to low-fat foods, balancing your plate is something you can do forever. Most people would find it unpleasant to eat mostly low-fat foods for a lifetime. But *balancing your plate*—always including some lower calorie foods on your plate—that's something you can do for the long term.

You'll eat more fruits and vegetables

Most people don't eat enough fruits and vegetables. If you're balancing your plate, the lower calorie options are going to be fruits and vegetables, so this will automatically help you eat more of them.

Slower eating

Finally, it'll slow down your eating. You'll balance the higher calorie, appetizing sandwich with the foods that are lower in calorie density (sliced fruits or vegetables, salad, or soup). You won't take seconds of whatever the main dish is, without finishing your sides.

Make the right choice convenient. Make the wrong choice inconvenient.

Years ago, before the obesity epidemic started, meals required planning. Fast food and other restaurants were uncommon. Grocery stores just carried ingredients, not full meals. Almost all foods required preparation at home. So, meals required at least some level of thought, ahead of time.

Times have changed. Now, the most delicious foods are available with a few clicks on a website. And there are convenience stores on every corner, that sell hundreds of different tempting junk foods.

As part of my research for this book, I was reading a memoir by a woman who had a life-long struggle with her weight. She'd been on many diets, and had chosen another one to try. On the first day of her diet, at 11:30 am (she had skipped breakfast), she ended up very hungry, browsing a food delivery website for options that would work for her. She ended up making a choice that she regretted, a heavy meal of Kung Pao chicken.

What led to this bad decision? Here's some of the factors:

- Powerful hunger pangs, after skipping a meal.
- Lack of planning
- The fact that she could, with one-click, order a very tempting, high-calorie meal online

Looking back, what are some of the things she could have done, in order to avoid this bad decision? She could have made the right choice convenient, and the wrong choice inconvenient.

The right choice would have been to bring lunch from home. It takes some planning and work to make this convenient. It means:

- Regular grocery shopping
- Having ingredients available in your kitchen.
- Prepping your lunch in the morning

The wrong choice was to buy a greasy, tempting, high-calorie meal from an online meal delivery service. She knew that this website was one that always tempted her to make bad choices. In theory, it would have been possible to order healthy foods, even on this website. But because the pictures of highly tempting, high-calorie choices were so overwhelming, she always ordered them.

Since our current food environment is so tempting, it makes sense to treat it as an enemy. You need to plan in advance to defeat this enemy. You need to make the worst options—such as this meal delivery website—impossible.

What could you do in this situation, to make the wrong choice more inconvenient? I suggest that you completely delete food delivery apps (Uber Eats, Seamless, and GrubHub) from your phone. Cross them off your list of options.

Some other ways of making the wrong food choices inconvenient are:

- Don't keep highly processed food/junk food in your home.
- Order groceries online from a list, if you're tempted by unhealthy foods when you're in the store.
- Leave your credit card at home. When you're spending cash instead of using a credit card, you're less likely to buy impulsively.
- Use personal food rules to make the wrong food choice inconvenient. For example, have a rule that you need to

make your own sweet snacks. That makes it less convenient.

And here's a few ideas for making healthy foods—the right choices—more convenient.

- Keep some healthy prepared foods around. For instance—hard-boiled eggs, string cheese, crunchy apples.
- Double up on familiar, healthy recipes. For instance, if you have a healthy chili recipe that you like, make double the normal recipe, and freeze the leftovers. That way you'll have a good option if you're short on time.
- Plan meals ahead of time. Find some default meal options that are healthy and convenient. Simple foods—like scrambled eggs or an omelet if you're rushed—are perfectly fine.
- Frozen foods are very convenient and easy, and you don't need to worry about them spoiling. Frozen berries are easy to add to smoothies and hot cereal. Frozen vegetables can be a quick and healthy side dish, to balance your plate.

Deciding at the last minute what you're going to eat usually leads to unhealthy choices. And relying on your willpower to avoid bad choices usually doesn't work.

It's best to take advantage of the times when you have willpower and energy, and *plan*. Plan how best to avoid your worst food habits. Figure out how to make the right choice convenient, and the wrong choice inconvenient.

Speaking of convenience and inconvenience—I reviewed a *lot* of diet books while researching this book. And I usually came across a "meal plan" section in the back, with something like this:

Week 1 Meal Plan - Breakfast
Day 1: Ricotta omelet and sweet potato hash browns
Day 2: Fall Pumpkin Oatmeal and strawberries
Day 3: Veggie Frittata with herbs and non-fat Greek yogurt
Day 4: Scrambled eggs with feta cheese and parsley
Day 5: Whole wheat toast with almond butter and banana slices
Day 6: Steel cut oats and non-fat Greek yogurt
Day 7: Blueberry-mango smoothie

These breakfasts sound tasty, but—what a lot of work! And this was just Week 1, breakfast. There was also the lunch, dinner, and snack plans, plus everything for weeks 2 through 4 as well, including the recipes. Some meals were repeated, but overall there were a tremendous number of recipes to learn, and prepare. And you would need loads of different ingredients for all the recipes.

If you had your own personal chef, this might be okay. But otherwise—this would not work for most people. It makes eating healthy too difficult. Yes, cooking and eating at home is best for managing your weight, but 7 *different* meals, just for Week 1 breakfast, makes things too inconvenient. Could you do this for a lifetime? I doubt it.

Have a mini-meal when necessary

What is a mini-meal? It's an acknowledgment that you don't always need to eat a "regular" meal, three times a day. It's saying to yourself, "I had an oversized lunch, now I'll have a very light dinner".

I'll give you an example. I was on a vacation with the whole family recently, and we went out to a restaurant for lunch. It was a small local restaurant, one that I'd never been to, and not part of a chain.

I'm normally careful when I eat at restaurants, so I looked carefully at the whole menu. I decided that the omelet was the best option. It came with toast, fruit, and french fries, but I substituted cottage cheese for the fries.

When the food came out, the omelet turned out to be enormous! It was delicious, but there must have been 4 eggs in it. And it had lots of cheese. The bowl of cottage cheese was massive. I could have made a meal just with the cottage cheese and toast alone.

Since we were traveling, I didn't want to bring leftovers to the hotel. And I have a really hard time leaving food on the plate. This is a bad habit to have at restaurants, incidentally.

So, I ate most of it, maybe leaving about one-third of the food behind. I felt uncomfortably stuffed afterward.

I'm usually hungry for my dinner at around 6. But that day, since I had a massive lunch, I wasn't hungry at all. The rest of the family was. So, while they ate, I just had a mini-meal—an apple and a slice of cheese. And that worked out just fine. I did get a little hungry later on in the evening, but it wasn't serious, so I just waited until breakfast.

Other options for mini-meals are a half slice of toast with a glass of milk, or a hard-boiled egg. Or perhaps a small bowl of light soup. Consider making the mini-meal under about 200 calories.

My normal rules and guidelines for restaurants would be:

- Eat at restaurants only occasionally.
- When I do eat at restaurants, I have standard meals, at restaurants that I know.
- If my meal is too large, I bring some of it home in a take-out container.

These usually work well—but not always. For instance, when you're traveling. When you're not at home, you eat at restaurants much more often. You don't necessarily know the restaurant, or what meals work well. And you can't bring any leftover food home with you.

But even if your regular food rules don't work, you can still manage your weight by using mini-meals.

And another important thing to mention is that—I could *easily* have eaten dinner that evening. No, I wasn't hungry, and I didn't need to eat, but it was mealtime. I wasn't overly full from lunch anymore. The rest of the family was eating. It would have felt comfortable to eat along with everyone else.

What made me choose to have a mini-meal instead? Yes, you guessed it—I knew I was going to weigh myself the next morning. We were traveling, so I had packed my travel scale. Having a regular meal on top of a huge meal would have caused a jump in my weight, which I didn't want to see. So, I had a mini-meal, and it worked out fine.

Weighing yourself daily makes these types of situations noticeable. But not weighing yourself daily makes them invisible. You're still gaining weight, but you're surprised by it. You wonder what happened.

Keep on weighing yourself daily.

Eat more slowly

I hesitated to include the guideline "Eat more slowly". It's a guideline that I don't find very easy to do myself. When I'm hungry, and there's a meal in front of me, I tend to eat quickly and steadily until it's all gone.

But still—even trying to eat a *little* more slowly is valuable, and here's why. It takes a *long* time for hunger to be satisfied, and a feeling of fullness to replace hunger. It's probably much longer than you think. Current studies show that it takes at least 20 minutes before your stomach catches up with what you've eaten.

What does this mean? Say you have a large meal in front of you, and you eat it quickly—in about 10 minutes. Since your stomach hasn't caught up with your eating, you're still feeling hungry. You'd start to feel full in another 10 minutes or so if you stopped eating. But instead, you serve yourself seconds, and continue eating.

About 30 minutes in, you're done. Your stomach has completely caught up, but now, instead of feeling comfortably full, you feel unpleasantly bloated. You wish you hadn't eaten so much.

Because of this delay before your hunger goes away, it's very easy to overshoot, and continue eating. Instead of getting to full, you're overfull. If you're eating a salad, this is not a problem. However, if you're eating something higher calorie, getting

263

uncomfortably full leads to many excess calories. And over time, that means weight gain, or having a harder time losing weight.

Eating quickly appears to be linked to obesity. That's something that makes sense, intuitively. But does eating quickly actually *cause* obesity? I don't think so.

I'm more inclined to think that there's a natural inclination some people have, which is a stronger-than-average drive to eat. And it's this inclination—the stronger-than-average drive to eat—that contributes to the tendency towards obesity, *and* the tendency to eat more quickly.

✳✳✳

There's a few techniques you can try if you'd like to eat more slowly. There are special forks, which will buzz if you take bites very quickly. Some people recommend that you use baby spoons, or chopsticks to slow down your eating. And many years ago, there was even a popular movement, promoting the idea that each bite you take should be chewed at least 32 times. Famous people of that era that gave it a try included John D. Rockefeller and Thomas Edison.

But...I just don't think consciously and deliberately slowing down your eating works, over the long term. Your pace of eating is more like your pace of breathing—not something that can be easily controlled.

Here's what can help. Just the knowledge that it takes a *long time* for feelings of fullness to develop—this is very useful. It can encourage you to wait a little, before serving yourself seconds. Also, balancing your plate with some lower calorie foods will help slow down your eating.

Bring food with you

Do you get hungry when you're out and about, and buy unhealthy snack food? Or maybe you have unplanned, impulsive, and unhealthy meals at restaurants because you get hungry?

If this is *not* you, then feel free to skip this section.

If it is, then consider this food guideline—*Bring food with you.*

You may ask—how does this help? If I always have food with me, aren't I more tempted to eat it? Well, yes. But consider the alternatives. If the alternative is to buy junk food from convenience stores, then a planned snack is much better. If you eat healthy foods you brought with you, instead of an impulsive restaurant meal, that's a much better choice.

Let's just be clear what "Bring food with you" does *not* mean. It does *not* mean highly processed foods like protein bars, energy bars, etc. It does *not* mean fruit snacks "made with 100% juice".

It means some almonds or peanuts. Or maybe an apple, and a slice of cheese. You want to have something basic, just in case you get too hungry. Not something that will tempt you to overeat.

If you're going to watch a movie at the theater, for instance, and normally buy candy or popcorn there—bring a little bag of dry roasted peanuts instead. Or make your own popcorn at home, and bring that.

A friend of mine, Brandon, started bringing food with him, when he was trying to lose weight. That was a great plan, *except* for one thing. The food that he was bringing with him was a bag of highly tempting, delicious smoked almonds. Smoked almonds are very easy to overeat, and they're very high-calorie. And it's not a good plan to always have tempting, high-calorie foods around.

Once he realized that he'd picked the wrong food, Brandon switched to plain raw almonds. They tasted okay to him, but they were not so tempting that he overate.

Plan for social events

Social events and gatherings—celebration meals at restaurants, potlucks, neighborhood block parties—can be tough when you're trying to manage your weight. The fact that there's all kinds of delicious foods available and everyone else is eating makes it extra hard.

You could decide that these types of events aren't enough of a problem for you to make specific plans. Maybe you know how much you generally eat at these events, and eating less the day before or the day after works for you.

For most people, though, these events can be a problem, and they need to really think about how to deal with them. Here's a few options that can help you limit the calories you consume:

Have only three items

If you're at a potluck or buffet, take a look at the food available. Figure out three items that would work for you, and only eat them. This gives you a lot of freedom, but also an upper limit, so that the variety doesn't become overwhelming.

Stick to your standard food rules

Say you have your standard food rules—for instance, *I make my own sweet snacks*. Don't make an exception because it's a special event. Stick to your rule. Especially if you have an upper limit rule for alcohol—say 2 drinks—keep to that maximum. If you overindulge in alcohol, that makes everything else harder to limit.

Eat before you go

Never go to a social event that involves lots of eating when you're really hungry. If you're famished and going to be faced with a huge variety of tempting foods, you probably won't make the decisions you should be making. Eat something before you go. Some cheese, a piece of fruit, even a small meal ahead eaten of time will help you avoid impulsive decisions.

Don't accept a plate with food on it

This happens a lot with celebration dinners. Maybe the host is being very efficient, and cutting dozens of large pieces of birthday cake. You stick out your hand when a plate is passed to you, and all of a sudden you own a large piece of cake, and feel like you need to finish it. Instead of doing this, realize—you don't need to accept it. Saying, "Not for me, thanks" is perfectly okay.

Summary

- If your rules aren't working, change them
- Variety is your enemy. Routine is your friend.
- One slice of bread instead of two.
- Hunger before meals is normal.
- Cook at home. Eat at home.
- Balance your plate.

- Make the right choice convenient. Make the wrong choice inconvenient.
- Have a mini-meal when necessary.
- Eat more slowly.
- Bring food with you.
- Plan for social events.

ONE LAST WORD

Keeping it up for a lifetime

At the end of most books on diet and weight management, there's a huge section with shopping lists and recipes. But this book doesn't have that.

It's not because I think recipes aren't useful—I look at cookbooks and recipes all the time. But this is not a diet book that says, "This is what you must eat, here's the foods you should buy, and this is the list of recipes". That approach is both too easy (no thinking involved, just do what you're told) and too hard (it's nearly impossible to keep up over the long term).

No, you need to figure out, mostly for yourself, what works and what doesn't. I have lots of suggestions in the chapters on food rules and guidelines. And there's plenty of information on what to be wary of in the chapters "Diet and Food Myths" and "Hazards You Need to Avoid".

I've tried hard in this book to convince to weigh yourself every single day. Being aware of and monitoring your weight is the cornerstone of losing it. And stepping on the scale every morning is essential if you want to keep the weight off long term. Please review the chapter "Why Weighing Yourself Daily is Essential" if you still have doubts. And when you come across the anti-scale messages that are so popular now, that tell you to "throw away your scale"—look carefully at where they're coming from. They're probably selling something.

Never forget that most people—more than 71 percent as of 2019—are overweight or obese currently. And that number is going *up*. People did *not* have more willpower 50 to 100 years ago, before everyone started gaining weight. They were not better people, and they did not have more self-control than we do today. No, the issue is that 100 years ago, people weren't faced with the extreme food temptations that we're now faced with every single day.

It's not possible to change the fact that tempting food is constantly available. But here's what *is* possible. You can:

- Understand the dangers of today's food environment, and how easy it is to gain weight.
- Weigh yourself daily.
- Develop your personal food rules, to reduce your food intake without needing willpower.

Thank you!

Thank you so much for reading Weigh Every Day. I hope it was useful for you, and that you now have a solid daily weigh-in habit, as well as some food rules that you've chosen for yourself.

If you were helped by this book, I'd really appreciate if you could write a review on Amazon. Most potential readers use reviews to decide whether to buy a book. And if you make progress in your weight loss goals, please mention that in your review as well. I'd love to hear what worked well, and what didn't. Every single review counts.

If you have comments on this book and would like to contact me personally, I'd be happy to hear from you. Feel free to send an email: Sylvia@WeighEveryDay.com.

For weight charts and other resources, blog posts, and contact information, please visit my website:

WeighEveryDay.com

NOTES

The History of Obesity

"more than 71% of the population is overweight or obese": Centers for Disease Control and Prevention, National Center for Health Statistics (September 2019), https://www.cdc.gov/nchs/data/hestat/obesity_adult_15_16/obesity_adult_15_16.pdf

"Katherine Flegal was a scientist at the Center for Disease Control": David A. Kessler, MD: The End of Overeating: Taking Control of the Insatiable American Appetite (New York, Rodale, 2009), 3.

"Statistics from the Center for Disease Control show that": Centers for Disease Control and Prevention, National Center for Health Statistics (September 2019), https://www.cdc.gov/nchs/data/hestat/obesity_adult_15_16/obesity_adult_15_16.pdf

"life expectancy has actually fallen in the United States": Murphy SL, Xu JQ, Kochanek KD, Arias E. Mortality in the United States,

2017. NCHS Data Brief, no 328. Hyattsville, MD: National Center for Health Statistics. 2018.

"But on the other hand, research shows us that some foods cause people to have very strong reactions": Marc Potenza et al., "Can Food be Addictive? Public Health and Policy Implications," Addiction 106, no. 7 (July 2011): 1208–1212.

"Many studies have shown that larger plates and bowls result in larger portion sizes": Brian Wansink et al., "Bottomless bowls: why visual cues of portion size may influence intake", Obesity Research 13 no. 1 (January 2005) 93-100.

"Humans behave the same as rats, when it comes to food variety": Kessler, p. 16.

"Some researchers claim that most of the extra calories that we're consuming these days come from snacks": Cutler, David, Edward Glaeser and Jesse Shapiro. 2003. "Why have Americans become more obese." Journal of Economic Perspectives 17, no. 3 (Summer 2003): 93-118.

"This fact was first discovered by Anthony Sclafani": Kessler, p. 15.

Why Weighing Yourself Daily is Essential

"More and more studies are coming out, showing that a daily weigh-in is strongly linked to weight loss.": Yaguang Zheng et al.,

"Self-weighing in weight management: a systematic literature review," Obesity (Silver Spring). 2015 Feb;23(2):256-65

"One study was done that compared two groups of overweight people": Dr Jessica LaRose et al., "Frequency of self-weighing and weight loss outcomes within a brief lifestyle intervention targeting emerging adults," Obesity Science & Practice, (2016 March) 88–92.

Diet and Food Myths

"a particular candy, when labeled as "fruit chew" was perceived": Irmak, Caglar & Vallen, Beth & Robinson, Stefanie. (2011). The Impact of Product Name on Dieters' and Nondieters' Food Evaluations and Consumption. Journal of Consumer Research. 38. 390-390. 10.1086/660044.

"people who were actively trying to lose weight ate more trail mix if it was labeled as a "fitness" snack": Koenigstorfer J, Baumgartner H: "The Effect of Fitness Branding on Restrained Eaters' Food Consumption and Post-Consumption Physical Activity". Journal of Marketing Research. 2016; 53 (1): 124-138.

Hazards You Need To Avoid

"There's a very clear relationship between eating restaurant food (including take-out and delivery food), and weight gain": Louis Goffe et al., "Relationship between mean daily energy intake and frequency of consumption of out-of-home meals in the UK National

Diet and Nutrition Survey," International Journal of Behavioral Nutrition and Physical Activity 14, no. 1 (September 2017)

"The Canadian Medical Association Journal published a report in 2017 which looked at 37 studies on artificial sweeteners.": Meghan B. Azad et al., "Nonnutritive sweeteners and cardiometabolic health: a systematic review and meta-analysis of randomized controlled trials and prospective cohort studies", Canadian Medical Association Journal 189, no. 28 (July 17, 2017): E929-E939

"According to a study in the British Medical Journal, wine glass capacity increased 7 times in the past 300 years.": Zupan Zorana et al., "Wine glass size in England from 1700 to 2017: a measure of our time", British Medical Journal 2017; 359 (December 13, 2017), j5623.

Food Rules—How They Can Work For You

"For instance, people eat a lot of candy if it's in a bowl right on their table": James E. Painter, Brian Wansink, and Julie B. Hieggelke, "How Visibility and Convenience Influence Candy Consumption," Appetite 38, no. 3 (June 2002): 237–38

Made in the USA
Las Vegas, NV
02 October 2024

96115412R10166